An Incredible
BOY
And A Remarkable
MAN

Ronald Stepp

ISBN 978-1-63844-253-0 (paperback)
ISBN 978-1-63844-254-7 (digital)

Copyright © 2021 by Ronald Stepp

All rights reserved. No part of this publication may be reproduced, distributed, or transmitted in any form or by any means, including photocopying, recording, or other electronic or mechanical methods without the prior written permission of the publisher. For permission requests, solicit the publisher via the address below.

Christian Faith Publishing, Inc.
832 Park Avenue
Meadville, PA 16335
www.christianfaithpublishing.com

Printed in the United States of America

ACKNOWLEDGMENTS

I would like to thank God for inspiring me to write this story of my brother Shelby and for guiding me from beginning to end. Also, I thank all my schoolteachers and Bible teachers who prepared me for learning throughout my life, especially Ms. Carrye Smith who taught me much more than arithmetic.

I am indebted to the other five Stepp boys, Rod, Butch, Jim, David, and Steve, who contributed facts about Shelby and experiences that they had with him that are a part of this book. I am especially grateful for Rod who remembered some things about Shelby that I had forgotten. Also, I appreciate the same type of contributions made by close friends Joe Hallford, Bill and Janice Hallford McFall, Jim Booher, Rita Allen, Mickey Aboussie, and a friend of Shelby's, Mary Weatherford Mock. My apologies to those of you who should have been added to this list, but that would have been a long, long list.

I was assisted voluntarily by the editing of the draft of each chapter by former high school classmate, Nancy White Ashbrook. She did a professional job and continuously offered me encouragement in completing this book. Finally, I thank Jeane, my wife of sixty years, for doing many chores for me during the fourteen hundred hours that I spent on this project.

Shelby's story is being told by his oldest brother, Ronnie, who was born one year, three weeks, and two days after him. To contrast Shelby's life with that of a normal baby, toddler, adolescent, teenager, and adult, much of the story is about Ronnie and their double cousin Rod.

PREFACE

In my eighty-three years, I have never met a more inspirational person than the one whose life story you are reading now. Shelby's life was a struggle from his first to his last breath, covering a period of almost sixty-nine years. Daily coping with multiple lifelong handicaps that quite possibly no other human has ever faced, his "can do" spirit and "do the best you can with what you have" attitude enabled him to accomplish more than anyone ever imagined.

Many of his family members, friends, and casual acquaintances of all ages, both living and deceased, have said that they were inspired by Shelby's life and that their lives were changed for the better because of him.

The first objective in writing his story is to inspire you and encourage you to achieve the ultimate in your short life here in preparation for living in eternity with God your Father and Jesus your Savior. The second objective is to enable you to genuinely feel that you knew Shelby. The third is that you will appreciate his mother's special loving care from his birth to adulthood until her death in September 1996. She was a Christian mother whose faith in God, love for her child, constant prayers for his life, and courage to endure all the negative aspects of his life were the ultimate testimony for all mothers. Finally, I pay tribute to Shelby's teacher as well as my teachers who gave us their best in bookwork and life experience and showed us how to be good citizens of strong character.

CHAPTER 1

Birth to Six Years (1936–42)

On April 8, 1936, Shelby Ray Stepp was delivered by Dr. George T. Singleton at the home of his parents, Lee Roy and Stella Ewing Stepp, at 2808 Lawrence Road, Wichita Falls, Texas. He was the first of four sons born to this couple, and they would have no daughters. Lee Roy and Stella were married in Wichita Falls on September 22, 1934.

For reasons never determined,[1] Shelby was born with cross-eyes[2] and without hands and feet,[3] but worse than those handicaps, he had no mouth.[4] Dr. Singleton quickly consulted with other local medical doctors about the newborn's absence of a mouth, and their consensus was that it would be most humane to let the baby die. His parents were informed of the key issues considered by the doctors in their deliberation of what could be done.

While his parents and Stepp's grandparents were considering their difficult decision, Grandma Stepp was rocking Shelby and noticed a small drop of saliva on his face at a site where a corner of his mouth would normally be. She then saw that the saliva was coming out of a pinhole. Mother began to feed her milk to him with an eyedropper through the pinhole. This method of feeding was continued for his first six months. Then Mother called Dr. Singleton and asked him to make an incision at the pinhole for a mouth opening. He said that it would be done as soon as possible.

An incision was made starting at the pinhole, creating an opening for Shelby's mouth. After a short period of healing, Dr. Singleton examined the inside of his mouth and noticed a one-inch tongue and underdeveloped jaw structures, which would preclude the growth of teeth. The smaller area of taste buds on his short tongue would limit his ability to taste. The amount of taste buds on the sides and back of his mouth was not determined. Thankfully, by the age of two, Shelby showed that he enjoyed eating and continued to do so for the remainder of his life.

The prognosis was that with lacking lips and having a nominal tongue, Shelby would not have the normal tools to speak or eat. Although the rim of his mouth looked much like lips, muscles were not present to manipulate the rim like a mouth. *These would prove to be his most severe handicaps.*

Obviously, Shelby would not be able to do most things that require the use of hands, and it would be difficult for him to walk and even more difficult to run or jump. A review of the list of things a normal person can do would show that Shelby would not be able to do hundreds of them. And with these apparent major physical handicaps, what if his mind was abnormal as well? What quality of life could Shelby have? What could he possibly do to make the world a better place?

Well, that is precisely what this story will tell you! Why did God allow such a fetus to live full-term? Be born?[5] Live almost sixty-nine years? Mother wrote the following when Shelby was about thirty years of age:

> They say that miracles don't happen, but Shelby is a living miracle. The doctors said that Shelby (at birth) couldn't live, but there isn't anything impossible with the Lord. Shelby seemed to be born with spunk and determination. With the Lord's help Shelby was able to overcome things that to you would seem impossible. He learned to walk without feet, to talk without a tongue, to write without hands. His greatest accomplish-

ment was to master the marimba which became his dearest way to serve the Lord. Though small, Shelby had great faith. He believed that the Lord could help and use him in many ways. The Lord blessed him with a sharp mind, and he was able to complete twelve grades of public school in ten years with high grades.

The questions above are answered in Mother's article. She revealed the core of Shelby's life story. The rest of his story that follows are the details of the same. As you continue reading, you will discover that Shelby was an incredible boy and a remarkable man who lived a life that inspired and encouraged thousands of others.

At six months of age, Shelby was the size of a normal baby of six weeks. He would always be undersized for his age because growth was impeded in his early years. With only one child, Mother had her hands full caring for Shelby because his needs increased as the months passed. She was holding him more and more of the time.

On May 2, 1936, Lee Roy's younger brother M. M. "Sonny" Stepp married Stella's younger sister Ruby Ewing Stepp. The two families began to share the house on Lawrence Road in early 1937. Shelby had his first birthday on April 8, 1937. On the same day, Uncle Sonny and Aunt Ruby had their first child and named him Roderick. He was Shelby's first double cousin and was called Roddy. His parents gave him no middle name but later asked him to pick his own. He chose David for his middle name.

On May 1, 1937, Mother and Daddy had their second son and named him Ronald Lee. He was called Ronnie. Roddy and Ronnie grew up much like twins.

In January 1938, the two Stepp families moved to a small house behind their Stepp Brothers Grocery store at 2206 Grant Street. Daddy and Sonny ran the store together for several years. In the early 1930s, Daddy had worked at a windows sash and door company and Long Bell Lumber Company in Wichita Falls. Sonny had owned a small café on Grant Street across from Sam Houston grade school.

He and Ruby lived in the back of the café until they moved in with Daddy and Mother and Shelby.

Stepp Brothers Grocery also included a manual gasoline pump (customers would hand-pump until the gasoline level in the glass cylinder reached the gallon mark they wanted), a manual dispenser of oil, a water hose, a kerosene tank, and an air compressor with hose and metal fitting. All of these were self-service for most customers. Also, they offered hamburgers, sandwiches, steaks, and other *home-cooked* food. A tall sign out near Grant Street read "Stepp Brothers Grocery-Service Station-Café." It also advertised "Hamburger 5 cents." Each year in season, black diamond watermelons from Rush Springs, Oklahoma, were lined up outside the immediate front of the grocery store.

The two Stepp families' three-room "shotgun" house served as a small duplex. The Lee Roy family's bedroom was on the south end, the Sonny family's bedroom was on the north end, and the two families shared the kitchen and dining room in the middle. The shared yard was about half grass and half dirt.

Shelby required a lot of Mother's time in his early years, so Ruby helped take care of Ronnie. Occasionally, Mother would take Ronnie to Grandpa Stepp's house, where Ronnie's aunt Lydia Stepp and cousin Dora Bond lived and left him in their care. Collectively, Mother, Ruby, Lydia, and Dora learned week to week and month to month how to best care for Shelby. For example, Mother discovered that she could not put his head under water without him choking. With no lips, he could not completely seal his mouth. But it was mostly Mother who cared for him from birth to age sixty. He required *so* much special care, some of which only she did for him.

On March 31, 1940, Uncle Sonny and Aunt Ruby had their second son and named him Michael Doyle. He was called Butch. Neither Rod nor Ronnie remembered who gave him that nickname, but it was about that time that Isaac Ewing gave Shelby his nickname Poofus. Uncle Ike was one of Mother's younger brothers. He was a real character who liked to "cut up" and "kid around," as did Poofus beginning early in his life. Uncle Ike could play the harmonica while driving a car with two hands on the steering wheel, accurately use a slingshot, and make up humorous nicknames for family and friends. Those talents and traits were very impressive to young boys. He and Poofus enjoyed each other for many years.

Ronnie's earliest memories of Poofus include seeing:

- Mother feed him little jars of Gerber baby food,
- him crawling around on his arm stubs and knees inside on the floor, and
- him sitting just inside the front screen door while watching Roddy and Ronnie playing outside, riding their tricycles and stick horses, running and jumping off the long front porch, and other things he could not do.

Ronnie's most vivid memory of Poofus is him doing his daily exercises. When he was about three years old, on his own, he developed a physical exercise routine that seemed to be precisely designed for him and which he performed daily. He would sit on the side of a bed or on a couch or in a chair with his legs hanging off and begin by extending his legs straight in front and scissor-kick rapidly about eight times, then just as rapidly roll his arms over and under each other horizontally in front of him (like "roll 'em up, roll 'em up, throw 'em in the pan") about eight times, then roll his head in a full circle once.[6] He would do about fifteen repetitions of this exercise each morning, and sometimes again in the afternoon or evening. And he continued doing them until late in life.

A memory of Poofus that was meaningful to Ronnie early in life was when he was four, Ronnie got to feed him Jell-O with a spoon. Even today, Ronnie has a vivid picture in his mind of sitting with Poofus at the small table next to the south window in the kitchen and dining room with Ronnie holding the spoon to Poofus's face. But he soon began to feed himself most of the time. He always wore a bib or something similar while eating.

In 1941, Lee Roy and Sonny had a home mover lift and rotate their house ninety degrees counterclockwise, and then they added three rooms to one side of the shotgun house with help from both Grandpas Stepp and Ewing. The three new rooms mirrored the three old rooms. What had been the single outside front door in the middle was now an inside door connecting the two kitchen and dining rooms. Lee Roy's family lived in the old rooms on the south while Sonny's family lived in the new rooms on the north. Roddy and Ronnie played mostly in the front yard, and Poofus often watched them riding their stick horses and tricycles and playing with toy cars and trucks while sitting inside his front screen door or in his rocker on the front porch.

About this time, Roddy and Ronnie had a real treat. They had their picture made in front of the grocery store while sitting on a pony with a pretty saddle. It became their lifetime favorite photo together. But five-year-old Poofus refused to be put on the pony.

On November 19, 1941, Poofus and Ronnie went to their first funeral, which was for Grandpa Robert Lee Stepp. That changed their lives in some ways. Eighteen days later, Japan attacked Pearl Harbor, and as with most people around the world, their lives changed in stages over the next four years. Mother was still carrying Poofus everywhere she took him. His small size enabled her to continue carrying him. Occasionally, she used a stroller. It was the "Hummer" of strollers.

Johna Huling Ewing, Mother's oldest brother, at age thirty-four, was a staff sergeant in the Second Battalion, Thirty-Sixth Division, Texas National Guard, when it was mobilized on November 20, 1940. The Thirty-Sixth Division participated in major US Army maneuvers in Louisiana in August–September 1941.

On November 21, 1941, the 2nd Battalion, 131st Field Artillery Regiment, 61st Field Artillery Brigade, 36th Division sailed from San Francisco for Brisbane, Australia. They stopped for supplies in Honolulu, Hawaii, on November 28 and left the next day for Brisbane. On December 7, they heard over the loudspeakers that Japan had attacked Pearl Harbor, and the United States was at war. After Christmas in Brisbane, the Second Battalion sailed again and arrived on the island of Java on January 11, 1942. During the Battle of Java, the Second Battalion distinguished itself fighting alongside Dutch, British, and Australian forces and would later be awarded a

Presidential Unit Citation. Uncle Johna was one of the first servicemen of the USA to fight in WWII.

However, the larger force of the Japanese continued to add manpower and superior weaponry, and on March 8, 1942, the Allies in the Dutch East Indies surrendered to the Japanese. Among the 32,500 soldiers taken prisoner, mostly Dutch, British, and Australian, were 534 members of the Second Battalion. Because there was nothing officially known about their fate until the end of the war, they were called "the Lost Battalion." Uncle Johna was a Japanese prisoner for three years and seven months. He spent much of his time working on the Burma Railway and the bridge over the River Kwai. Poofus, Roddy, and Ronnie had last seen him in early November 1941.

Ronnie does not remember anything about Christmas 1941 other than Poofus and he got robes and pajamas, and Ronnie also got "house shoes," while Poofus got wool stockings.

Other memories of Ronnie during Poofus's first five years include watching him:

- walking around on his knees instead of crawling (Mother often sewed patches at the knees of his long pants),
- riding on his toddler toy locomotive on Christmas Day 1940 with Uncle Ike helping him (Isaac Ewing would soon join the US Navy),
- playing with Ronnie's WWII army olive-drab painted truck with matching cover over the top frame behind the cab,
- catching and throwing a rubber ball,
- stacking wooden alphabet blocks,
- sitting or rocking in his rocking chair, and
- coloring in his coloring books with his Crayola crayons.[7] Poofus held a crayon the same as a pencil. Everything that Ronnie did with a thumb and index finger, he did with his two stubs. Their youngest aunt, two youngest uncles, and older cousins taught them to color and draw.

Some of Poofus's other favorite things to do during his first six years include the following:

- riding with Uncle John in his delivery truck (John E. Stepp was their dad's oldest brother); this was one of Poofus's favorite things to do even when he was ten years old
- visiting with four grandparents, ten aunts, ten uncles, fifteen cousins, and friends
- proudly seeing six uncles and three cousins going off to WWII
- listening to Mother reading children and Bible stories
- singing hymns and praises at church
- listening to Daddy playing "Under the Double Eagle" on his fiddle
- going to Grant Street Park at night to watch a free movie starring Tom Mix and others while sitting on a blanket
- sitting on the wooden produce stand outside Stepp Brothers Grocery Store beside the front door.

It was made of plywood and was four feet by four feet by four feet. From there, he could watch the comings and goings of customers and vehicle traffic on a busy Grant Street. During WWII, he often watched military convoys, sometimes for hours, going south to Houston to ship overseas. He spent a lot of time there until he was ten. For many people who came to know Poofus, that was where they first saw him.

All his life, people of all ages would react when they first saw Poofus. Children would sometimes show fear and cry. Some children would cringe and wrap their arms around their mom or dad or older sibling. Some adults did not know what to do or say. But Poofus made many lifelong friendships from early childhood and throughout his life. He had a good sense of humor and enjoyed kidding around with all ages.

At the back of the Stepp brothers' lot was a wood-framed washhouse with wood siding and a flat roof with a slight pitch. Inside in one corner was a toilet. Two walls had shelves, which were almost full of cigar boxes containing receipts and other paper records of Stepp Brothers Grocery. The two Stepp families bathed in a galvanized metal tub.

A small tree grew close to the washhouse, and when Roddy and Ronnie were age five, it was tall enough for them to climb from it on top of the roof of the washhouse. They could watch people walking down the alley without being seen. Most evenings, Mr. Woodward, who lived across the alley, would walk his dog several miles always beginning and ending down the alley. Many times, they heard him talking to his dog, and it caused them to giggle from atop the wash house, but he never noticed them. *Poofus could not join them on top of the building.*

During WWII, it was good to have a grocer in the family. They had ration books like everyone else, but they had first shot at items that were in short supply. To a boy of five to eight years that included Fleers Dubble Bubble gum, which was kept in the box it came in hidden under the counter. *But Poofus could not chew gum.*

Also, in 1942, Uncle Sonny started working at Wichita Engineering Company welding bomb casings, which were sent by rail to the first WWII bomb manufacturing plant in the USA. He worked there until WWII ended. In 1944, when some employees were being led by a union leader to strike, Uncle Sonny wrote an anonymous poem and letter to all employees stating his opposition to the strike. When he got to work the next day, he put it on the Wichita Engineering bulletin board. It said:

> The *Boss* is just a tight wad,
> "He's a crank" they say,
> As they gang up on "his time"
> To talk about 'his pay.'
> Yeah he's just a glutton__
> This is *CIO* talk,
> He's the meanest man they know,
> They even cuss his walk.
> But to me he seems quite different,
> Never seems to cause much fuss,

RONALD STEPP

He's done a lot for *Uncle Sam*,
And made good jobs for us.
No Sir, I ain't squawking,
And there's one thing I know,
That we won't speed up *V-day*
By joining the *CIO*;
So, if you say, "We'll forget the *Boss*
And show him no respect at all";
But turn our thoughts to the *G. I. Joes*
Who are doomed to fall.
While they are in there fighting
A battle hard we know,
We stand around on our jobs
And holler *CIO*.
Yeah, they're in there pitching,
Fighting like a blaze,
And they're not griping either
To get a nickel raise.
Then let's think of the *G. I.'s kiddies*
As they're told a story sad,
"Your *Dad* was killed in action,
But he gave them all he had."
So let's have cooperation
And show our respect to *"Joe"*
And vote against those troublemakers,
Namely, *CIO*.
Let's give 'em stuff to fight with
Until this battle's won.
That's doing very little
Compared to what they've done.
And as they fight to keep down trouble,
So they can come home soon,
Let's vote against the troublemakers
Tomorrow afternoon.
If you care to know this author,
Well, I'll tell you, gentlemen.

AN INCREDIBLE BOY AND A REMARKABLE MAN

He's in your midst and working,
And he wears a safety pin.

(Uncle Sonny placed this poem on a bulletin board of the Wichita Engineering plant in Wichita Falls, Texas, during WWII early in the morning of the day before the employees voted on a motion to go union. The majority voted *no*! This poem was circulated across the manufacturing plants of the USA to influence the vote of whether to go union.)

Many years later, Ronnie came up with a title for the poem:

Are You for CIO or G. I. Joe?
by M. M. "Sonny" Stepp

* * * * *

The two Stepp families shared a four-door sedan until 1944. The car was usually parked beside the store in front of their house. During World War II, deliveries of grocery store items were sometimes slow, so one of the four parents would go pick up some items downtown near the train depot. One time when they got back with a carload of groceries, Roddy and Ronnie got a carton of cigarettes out of the car, opened a pack, got a cigarette each, got some matches, and tried to light the cigarettes. They would not burn, so they would throw them away and try to light two more. They did this again and again but could never get one to burn.

Although older than us, *Poofus never misbehaved like us at this time in his life.*

There was an Amur River privet bush in their backyard next to the Hallford fence. Chester and Faye Hallford lived next door. They had a daughter, Janice, who was two years younger than Poofus. The privet bush was perfect for easily getting a three-foot slender branch that was good for whippings. Most of the branches were the right size. They were readily available to their parents from 1938 to 1944. They stung like fire when used on bare legs, but they did not bruise them. Mother and Daddy never had to go to the privet bush because of Poofus. In Ronnie's opinion, Uncle Sonny and Aunt Ruby should have gone there more often.

When Poofus was four, Roddy or Ronnie

- poured sand in the two-family car gas tank,
- opened the small metal lid of the underground gasoline tank and dropped gravel one pebble at a time into it just to hear the unique sound when it hit the bottom, and
- filled his cowboy hat with kerosene and then drank it like Tom Mix.[8]

(The privet bush was tapped quite a few times.)

Mother began to replace baby food for Poofus with the meals she prepared for her family. She would crumble hamburger meat and chop up pieces of beef cutlet, beef roast, fried chicken, pork chop, ham, and meat loaf into tiny pieces. She would mash fruit and vegetables and desserts. All his food was somewhere between pureed and mashed. He loved mashed hot tamales and Wolf brand chili and ice cream (this one by itself). Food became more and more important to Poofus, and he enjoyed eating. *And he was always feeding himself now with a fork or spoon or glass.*

When Poofus was five, Roddy and Ronnie did the following:

- Rode their tricycles through very cold ponds of water at the Grant Street and Cumberland Street intersection, went into their house, turned on the gas to a space heater by Ronnie's small bed, got a match from the kitchen, struck the match at the gas heater. *Poof!* Ronnie's blanket caught fire, but they were quickly rescued. The privet bush donated two more branches.
- Found some rolls of Indian Head Pennies in the wash house, took some out by the alley, unrolled them, and threw a lot of them into Mr. Woodward's flower garden. (Mr. Woodward was principal at Austin grade school where Poofus would later complete all twelve grades in a special education class.

Neither he nor his wife ever invited them into their yard, much less their house.) Another two-brancher.

- Were in the wash house at the back of their lot, and Roddy asked for Ronnie's boots. Ronnie took them off and gave them to Roddy. Ronnie started climbing the wall shelves to see what was in some of the newer cigar boxes. Meanwhile Roddy spread toilet paper all over the wooden floor and then struck a match and lit the paper. Ronnie smelled smoke, looked down, saw the floor on fire, and remembered that he was barefoot. Thankfully, Roddy had a change of heart and ran to get his mother who rescued Ronnie. No whipping for Roddy; Aunt Ruby thought he had suffered enough emotionally. Ronnie thought a privet branch whipping was required.

- "Stole" a little box of candy-coated chewing gum with Feen-a-Mint[9] on the label, went out the store's front door to the north side of the store, sat down, and chewed several pieces each. Soon thereafter, they ran to the wash house.

- "Stole" fudgesicles while a tall stack of boxed grocery items shielded the ice cream box from their dads' view. They ate them while playing in their backyard. Ronnie ate his quickly while playing. Roddy wanted to make his last longer, so he kept taking a bite, putting the fudgesicle under a bedroom pillow, playing a while, taking a bite, etc. until it was all eaten.

- Each took an ice pick stuck in a wood shelf of canned goods next to the *Coca-Cola* icebox, went out the store's front door, and bombed Tojo's[10] Japanese ships (black diamond watermelons). About a dozen customers got free melons. (Yep, two-brancher.)

When Poofus was six, Roddy and Ronnie did the following:

- Climbed up the hog wire fence between the Stepps and the Hallfords, stood on top of the fence with their arms

wrapped around a bunch of cane stalks, pushed off forward, and rode the stalks down to the ground.
- Climbed on top of the wash house and threw their lightweight balsa planes as high as they could and repeated that many times.
- Climbed on top of the roof of the air compressor building roof, then up on the grocery building roof, and walked over onto the flat roof above the gas pump.
- Got six empty soft drink bottles from the grocery store's wood cases of empties and went to Mr. Hudgen's store one block away and told him their dads wanted to exchange them for a plug of Brown Mule chewing tobacco. He took their bottles and gave them the tobacco. They went to one corner of Grant Street Park, got behind some tall bushes, and Ronnie took a chew. After swallowing too much of the juice, his legs got weak and his stomach got to churning. Ronnie spit out the tobacco. Roddy never took a bite. Mr. Hudgins knew what he was doing and what they were doing.

Note how much of this and the prior page coverage is about Roddy and Ronnie and how little is about Poofus. That is a legitimate measuring stick of the physical activities of a normal child age three to eight versus those of Poofus at the same age. And that differential remained similar for five more years.

Poofus still needed Mother to bathe him, button his shirts, roll up his long sleeves, zip or button his pants, snap his suspenders, comb his hair, and assist him in the restroom. Also, from age five to eight, she pinned a handkerchief to the front of his shirt or bib overalls so he could wipe saliva, which often drooled from his mouth. She replaced it several times each day. He drooled all his life.

At this point in his life, Poofus had never done anything bad like Roddy and me. He spent most of his time in his rocker in the backyard or on the front porch watching us. And he spent almost as much time sitting on the produce box watching whatever. Together that adds up to most of his day.

What were his thoughts? Would he ever be able to do what he saw Roddy and Ronnie doing? Drive a truck like Uncle John? His daddy walked on his hands all the way around the outside perimeter of the duplex. Would he ever be able to walk around it on his stubs? Somehow, God enabled Poofus to be content with his life, keep a positive attitude, and develop a good sense of humor. God must have used Mother to accomplish that. He certainly did not use Ronnie or Daddy.

By now it was obvious to Mother that Poofus was not mentally impaired, and she was most grateful to God for that fact. Ronnie never gave that any thought until he met "Judge," who was a young man who often walked by the grocery store dressed in blue denim bib overalls. Ronnie soon found out that he was mentally impaired and felt sorry for him.

A few years later, Roddy and Ronnie occasionally saw a young man who lived on Grant Street, one block south of their home, and it became apparent to them that he was mentally impaired. His name was Myron Hurst, and Ronnie found a Bible at HHBC on a Sunday night that had his name in it. Ronnie took it to Myron's house and returned it to him. Ronnie felt sorry for Myron, but he does not remember ever feeling sorry for Poofus because of his handicaps.

One big plus for Poofus was the large number of aunts, uncles, and cousins that were living in the Wichita Falls area. They were two large, loving, caring families, most especially for Poofus. He got more attention than any other and required and deserved it. From Ronnie's personal experience with many of them, both the Stepps and the Ewings, all of the Stepp boys got a lot of help and support in their formative years. All ages of them helped in all aspects of their lives. Some of them were instrumental in their preschool (at home) preparation for the early grades of public school.

In their early years, Aunt Era Stepp Bond and her family and Aunt Lydia Stepp lived with Grandpa and Grandma Stepp at 2714 Pennsylvania Road. Grandpa Stepp had built the house in the late 1920s. Their lots were a half block from the western edge of town. Aunt Lydia and Cousin Dora "Punkie" Bond were good babysitters. Lydia was Punkie's aunt too, but she was only one year older than Punkie. Sometimes Mother would take Poofus and Ronnie over there and visit. Punkie often played music on an electric record player. *Poofus really enjoyed that.*

Grandpa Stepp had built a storm cellar between the house and garage. Mother and Ruby took the five Stepp boys over there three or four times when a tornado warning was in effect. The first time they went in the cellar, Grandma Stepp churned butter while Poofus, Roddie, and Ronnie watched. Grandpa Stepp always had a large vegetable garden and some fruit trees. Also, he raised chickens and pigs and had a milk cow. Although Poofus, Roddy, and Ronnie were "city slickers," they got to see a hog killed, cleaned, butchered, and some of the pork served at mealtime the same day. Also, they saw chickens killed by having their necks wrung. They thought it was fun to see them flopping around violently without a head.

Adjoined to his garage, a woodwork shop of Grandpa Stepp was found, and he was always making furniture for family members in the 1920s and 1930s. One is a checker or chess table made of light and dark wood with attractive grain and border. In 1940, he built a large room at the back of his house for Punkie and her husband, Ernest Johnston. Often, he worked as a carpenter and painter around town. He had no car during his last several years, so Poofus and Ronnie would often go with Mother to take him to a job and pick him up when he was ready to go home. But they did not get to know him very well because of their young ages.

Aunt Era's two youngest sons, Alvin and Charles Ray Bond, were five and three years older than Roddy and Ronnie. Alvin and Charles treated them well most of the time, but when Roddie and Ronnie were five years old, they often scared them with tales of the Frankenstein monster and the Wolfman, and they came out of hiding in Grandpa Stepp's dark garage, sneaked up behind them, and hollered loudly. Also, Alvin and Charles taught them to say cuss words. They never did these things to Poofus, and neither did Roddy and Ronnie.

On most Sundays in the 1940s, after church and lunch, Mother and Ruby would take Poofus, Roddy, Butch, and Ronnie to Grandpa Eddie Lee and Grandma Essie Almeda Ewing's home in the country south of town. Usually, three or more of the families, Mother's siblings, would be there. The kids played outside while the adults visited inside. Most had been to Sunday school and worship service,[11] but Grandpa usually preached or taught a Bible lesson to the adults while the children played. Poofus sat in a rocker on the front porch and watched them.

The Ewing house sat on a hill north of Lake Wichita that had an irrigation ditch with slow flowing water that the kids could play in or near depending on their ages. They also had a cotton patch, and Ronnie picked cotton with Uncle Ike one time when he was five, but he quit after thirty minutes. *Poofus did not pick or pull a single boll.* But he enjoyed sitting on the high front porch and watching the nearby windmill turn and the chickens and guineas grazing. *They always had at least one mean bantam rooster that chased Ronnie but never Poofus.* Later they moved closer to the lake. Neither place had plumbing or electricity.

In 1943, they moved to a house in town with plumbing and electricity on Baltimore Road. After several moves in a short period, they ended up on Colquitt Road, and the Sunday visits continued as did Grandpa Ewing's preaching and teaching. At that time, Colquitt Road was the western boundary of residences in that part of town. They lived there until Grandpa died in 1961. In 1933, he was one of the last electric streetcar drivers in Wichita Falls when the streetcars quit running late in that year. He then worked most of the time as a carpenter.

On their living room wall was a card, which read:

> Only one life, 'twill soon be past, Only what's done for Christ will last.[12]

From time to time for over seventy years, Ronnie has quoted it and mentioned it to others, but he does not remember talking about it to Poofus.

Because their extended family encouraged them, Roddy and Ronnie were always at the top of their classes at Sam Houston grade school in reading, spelling, and arithmetic, and in writing, they were above average. *Later, when Poofus went to school, he was also at the top of his classes.*

Until he was eight, Poofus was often watching what Roddy and Ronnie were doing, but he remained innocent of improper behavior, and as far as they know, he never tattled on them. However, in most cases, their parents found out somehow.

Our Christmas 1942 gifts were mostly clothes. Because WWII was in full swing, items made of metal and rubber were in short supply for civilians, and that included most toys. Poofus got shirts, pants, coat, suspenders, and a metal toy pickup with side boards like Uncle John's. Ronnie got a blue Navy officer uniform with a cap and leather Sam Browne belt and shoulder strap, shoes, bib overalls, shirts, and a cap gun.

With Mother's loving care and the grace of God, Poofus was healthy during his first six years. Ronnie took that for granted then, but he is amazed now.

Before going to the seventh year of Poofus, it must be noted that Roddy had several match-striking incidents in neighbor A. B. Hall's dry grass backyard.

* * * * *

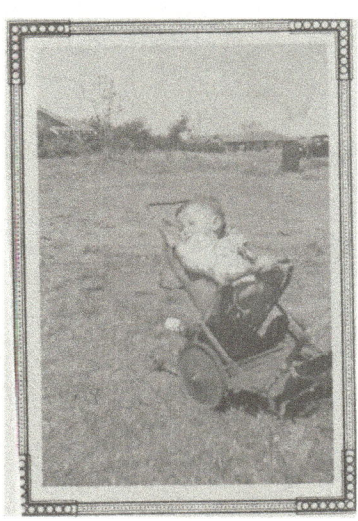

Shelby at age two in front yard

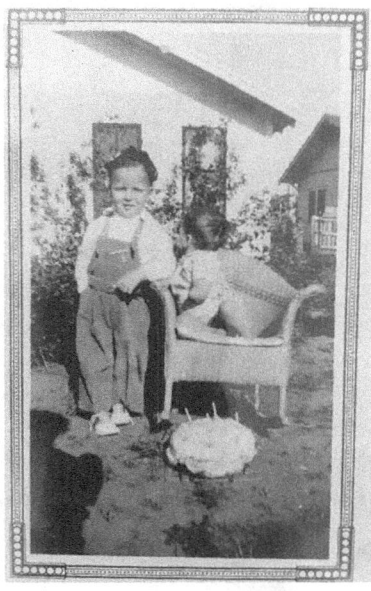

Ronnie and Shelby on Shelby's 4th BD

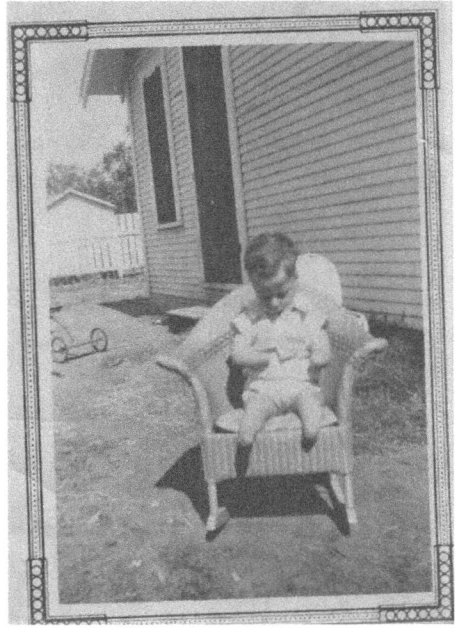

Back yard on his 4th birthday at 2206 Grant Street

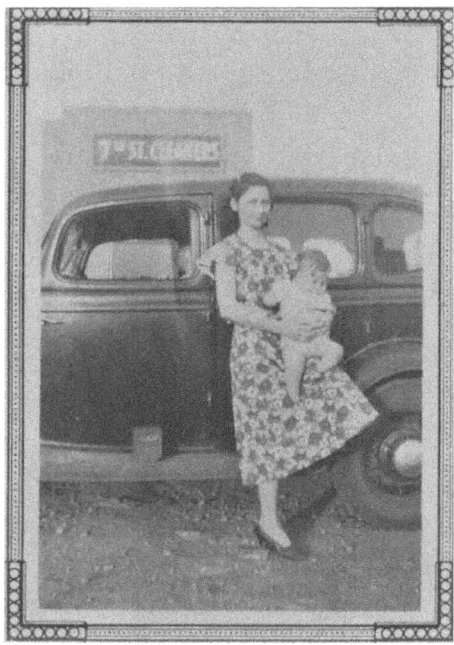

Stella holding Shelby in 1937

---

[1] The first thalidomide-affected baby was born in West Germany in 1956. Babies have been born with impairments like those caused by thalidomide throughout history.

[2] About 3 percent of children in the United States have crossed eyes after age one.

[3] December 05, 2019—CDC estimates that each year, about 1,500 babies in the United States are born with upper limb reductions and about 750 are born with lower limb reductions. In other words, each year, about 4 out of every 10,000 babies will have upper limb reductions, and about 2 out of every 10,000 babies will have lower limb reductions. Statistically, only 1 out of 12.5 million would have both impairments. In 2018, the number of babies born in the United States was 3,788,235. In 1936, the number of babies born in the USA was 2,144,790.

[4] Research found zero newborns without a mouth in the USA. Statistically, only one baby would be born in the United States in multiple centuries with all of Shelby's impairments.

5. The reader may find it helpful to do this exercise to get the feel of what it did physically for Poofus. He could rapidly move his shorter legs with no weight beyond his stubs.
6. "'Neither this man nor his parents sinned,' said Jesus, 'but this happened so that the work of God might be displayed in his life'" (John 9:3).
7. The reader can relate to the challenge this activity presented to Poofus by placing a crayon or pencil on a table with a tablet. Pick the crayon up using your two fists. Roll it between the two fists until the pointed end of the crayon can contact the tablet. Start coloring.
8. Ronnie was Tom Mix.
9. A chewing gum laxative.
10. They learned later that they should have bombed Admiral Yamamoto's ships because Tojo commanded the Japanese Army. One of their older cousins or uncles should have corrected them. In any case, the customers got free melons.
11. Mother and Aunt Ruby started taking their sons to Sunday school and worship at two months of age. Ronnie does not know when Mother started taking Poofus, but it was before Ronnie was born. Uncle Sonny went most of the time, but Lee Roy did not go much at all until 1952.
12. Written by Charles T. Studd, English missionary who faithfully served His Savior in China, India, and Africa from 1910 to 1931.

CHAPTER 2

Seven to Twelve Years (1943–48)

At the age of seven, Poofus began to learn how to do more of the things that Roddy and Ronnie were doing (the good things). Using his vocal cords, short tongue, and throat muscles as best he knew how, he could now speak well enough for Mother and Ron to understand most of what he said. Aunt Ruby and Roddy could understand him to a lesser degree. Most people could not understand what he said.

By this time, Poofus and Ronnie had said goodbye to Uncle Johna Ewing (Army), Uncle Isaac "Ike" Ewing (Navy), Cousin William "Buddy" Bond (Coast Guard), Cousin Paul "Tinesy" Bond (Navy), Uncle Willie "Bud" Ewing (Marines), Uncle Mabry Erwin (Army), and Uncle Roy Mansell (Army) as they left to fight in WWII. Mabry was the husband of our aunt Ruth Ewing Erwin. Roy was the husband of our aunt Almeda Ewing Mansell.

Uncle Bud Ewing was one who helped Poofus and Ronnie learn to use crayons. He enlisted in the US Marines several months before he turned seventeen on February 15, 1943. He lied about his age, and his parents signed the papers. Not only was he underage, but he was small for his age. His recruiting sergeant must have seen the grit in him. Ronnie remembered a few days before Uncle Bud went overseas, he took Roddy and Ronnie to Grant Street Park and showed them how to swing hand by hand across the "monkey bars."

AN INCREDIBLE BOY AND A REMARKABLE MAN

Although there was no official word of the whereabouts of "the Lost Battalion," they were believed to be prisoners of Japan. Uncle Bud said he was going to free his brother Johna (not a misprint) when his Marines got to Japan. He later got as close to Japan as Okinawa, which is 385 miles from the southern tip of Japan. However, Johna was probably still in Thailand, which is about 2,000 miles from Okinawa. Bud was awarded the Purple Heart when he was wounded in the back by shrapnel. That wound bothered him all his life. He became a career Marine and fought later in Korea. He wrote to Poofus, Rod, Butch, and Ronnie from overseas occasionally.[1]

On August 18, 1943, Uncle Sonny and Aunt Ruby had their third son and named him James Lesley. He was called Jim.

Two weeks later, Rod and Ronnie started first grade in public school. There were two classes for each of the six grades, but Rod and Ronnie were in Mrs. Ruth Watson's class. They brought books and other materials home, and Poofus began to look through them. As their school year progressed, Shelby accumulated a lot of basic awareness of learning. He learned to page through the soft-covered readers (*Dick and Jane, Tom, Tip and Jane,* etc.) by holding the left page down with his left stub (which was just below his elbow, large and round) while pushing the right page to the left with his right stub (which was where his wrist should be, smaller and pointed). As with everything else Poofus learned, it was all trial and error and try to do it better and faster next time. Sometimes he got frustrated with himself, but he soon restarted his "can do" attitude.

Cousins Alvin and Charles taught Rod and Ronnie how to make a kite with sticks from Grandpa's wood scraps, newspaper, homemade paste, flour sack scraps for the tail, and string. And they taught them how to fly it. Also, they taught them how to shoot a single-shot .22 rifle and how to handle it safely. And they taught them how to play the game of marbles. Rod and Ronnie had a flat area of dirt with no grass near their alley to play marbles. They only competed against each other. The most important part of the game is shooting a marble from your hand with the flick of your thumb, knocking a marble out of the circle, while leaving your shooter marble in the circle. Poofus could not make a kite or shoot a .22 rifle or play marbles, but he could fly a kite.

Uncle Harry "Boydie" Ewing, the youngest sibling of their mothers, was three years older than Poofus. He visited them frequently and played with Poofus, Rod, and Ronnie. He also took up for them. One day he came to see them and saw Johnny Bridges and Gene Leach, two years older and much bigger than Roddy and Ronnie, picking on them. He fought them and ran them away. Gene later shot Rod in the back of the head with his BB rifle while they were walking by his house. He may have been aiming for Ronnie. Nobody ever bothered Poofus, but that was little consolation for his handicaps.

Boydie also taught Rod and Ronnie to stomp down on the middle of two empty oil cans, one for each foot, which would result in both ends of the cans clamping around the sides of their shoes. Then they could walk around the concrete pavement of the filling station or grocery store and make a lot of noise. Poofus never did that even after he learned to walk because he was too old for that.

One day Rod and Ronnie walked six blocks to a house on Wenonah Boulevard that was having a garage sale. Each bought a thin metal hen that laid an egg when you pushed her body down her legs to the feet. The egg was a marble. They worked every time. Poofus liked Ronnie's so much that he gave it to him.

On October 2, 1943, Poofus went to his second funeral, which was for Grandma Sarah Isabel Kelly Stepp. It was held in HHBC and was very meaningful to him and to Ronnie. She was a good grandma to the Stepp boys. Three days earlier, Rod and Ronnie were in school when they were told by Mrs. Watson that their grandma Stepp had died and that they were to leave school immediately and walk to her house. They walked twelve blocks by themselves[2] to her house.

Daddy splurged and bought a nice big console radio. Poofus and Ronnie began to listen to music and *The Lone Ranger* on the radio. Mother listened a lot each day while she did her housekeeping and family chores. She had many favorite morning radio shows, but Ronnie only remembers *Stella Dallas* and *Just Plain Bill*.

AN INCREDIBLE BOY AND A REMARKABLE MAN

Christmas morning of 1943, Rod excitedly told Ronnie that he had seen Santa Claus bring in their presents. Ronnie was disappointed that he had not been awake to see Santa, but he felt good about obeying his parents by not peeking. Some years later, Rod told Ronnie that he had lied about that. Of course, Ronnie knew by 1945 that Rod had lied. On Christmas Day, Daddy moved his family two blocks north to 2804 Avenue L. Poofus got a toy six-shooter with a holster, and Ronnie got a Lincoln Logs set, and they both got Bible storybooks with pictures. Ronnie could shoot caps in his cowboy revolver, but Poofus could only hold his gun and point it.

Living on Avenue L placed Ronnie in the Crockett grade school district, but Mother went to the Crockett office and applied for permission for him to continue attending Sam Houston grade school. Permission was granted.

Soon Mother began taking Poofus and Ronnie to a movie theater on Monroe Street almost every week. Early on it was called the Roxy theater and later the Linda theater. Often, they would see Roy Rogers, Gene Autry, or another cowboy movie star. Then they would go home; put on their cowboy hat, gun, and holster; and act out the movie. Ronnie would provide the sounds and background music, and Poofus would energetically join in the shooting and fisticuffs or stubicuffs.

Ronnie has a list on a school form signed by Mrs. Watson of the twenty-nine books he read in the first grade. Poofus heard him read many of them, and he stubbed through most of them. Their mothers got one subscription to *Child Life* magazine for the four Stepp boys to share. Poofus enjoyed finding the "hidden objects." They got *Child Life* for many years because of Butch and Jim.

Uncle Louis Watkins entered the Air Force on June 6, 1944 (D-Day), and made it to the Marianas, but by that time, the war was almost over. Louis was married to Aunt Lydia Stepp Watkins, our Lee Roy's youngest sister. They were among the favorite aunts and uncles of Poofus and Ronnie. Cousin Lesley "Scrootch" or "Clem" Bond joined the Navy, but he spent most of his active duty in Washington state maintaining Navy airplanes with pontoons.

In July 1944, when Poofus was eight, the M. M. Stepp family moved about seventeen blocks to 2814 Lawrence Road. Ronnie spent the night with them in early August, and after breakfast the next morning, Rod and Ronnie walked to Ronnie's house and got the surprise of their lives. When they walked into the living room, Poofus got up and walked over to them on his stubs on the large rug. He then walked from the couch across the rug to a club chair. Then he walked between the chair and couch repeatedly as Rod and Ronnie watched with amazement. Of course, Poofus was more thrilled than they were.

Being able to walk changed his life forever.

About a month later, Mother went to a local boot maker and talked to the cobbler about making shoes with round soles for Poofus. Lace-up shoes were made for him, which became another activity for someone to do for him. His right leg was almost an inch shorter than his left, which required a layer of soft leather between the inside cushion and the sole of the right shoe. During the following years, the boot maker improved the shoe design and materials as Poofus outgrew them or wore them out.

The Christmas 1944 was a another good one for Poofus and Ronnie. Since he could now walk, he could wear long pants and not wear out the knees. He got a new cowboy hat, a pair of Levi's, a cowboy vest and shirt, books, and a three-fourths-size toy army rifle, which looked like a real one. Ronnie got clothes, an army rifle, and a bow and arrow set with rubber cups on the target end of the arrows. Poofus could only watch Ronnie shoot arrows, but they often played army.

Poofus and Ronnie often listened to *Fibber McGee and Molly*, *Amos and Andy*, and *The Lone Ranger* on the radio. Now, Poofus expected Mother to take them to a movie every week. And she did take them most weeks. The movies were often about WWII, so they learned how to fight the Germans and Japs, which they did a lot in their backyard. They played together more since Rod moved. *Ronnie could stand and run while playing with Poofus now instead of playing with him on his knees. And they talked to each other much more now, and Ronnie began to understand him as well as Mother did.*

After school, Ronnie often watched the sixth-grade boys play softball games against other grade school teams. He remembers two brothers who were good pitchers for Sam Houston. They were Charley and Johnny Deal. Each following year, he watched the softball games and learned the rules of the game and how to pitch, hit, field, and run the bases.

In April 1945, Ms. Eula Hardeman, Ronnie's second grade teacher, took her class to Grant Street Park for an Easter egg hunt. Poofus watched them from his front porch across the street. Poofus got to participate a few days later in two egg hunts. One was at HHBC and the other was at Uncle Johnny and Aunt Laverne's farm in Wichita Valley Farms in the annual Ewing family egg hunt. *Because he could now walk, this was his first year to hunt Easter eggs without help from others.*

Ms. Hardeman also taught her class to square dance during the current school year. At the end of the school year, she picked four boys and four girls to go to other schools to perform during their third grade year. Ronnie got picked for next year. Rod had Ms. McKinney for second grade teacher and did not get to learn square dancing, but he liked his teacher. When playing softball during recess, Ronnie was often the pitcher. Cousin Charles gave him an old ball glove and bat. *But Poofus could not play softball at this time.*

In June 1945, Ronnie made a profession of faith in Jesus Christ as his Savior and Lord during Vacation Bible School. He remembers walking home from Highland Heights Baptist Church with Mother. She was a VBS teacher. It was only a seven-block walk, and they were talking about the decision he had just made. Today Ronnie can vividly picture in his mind walking across Grant Street Park with Mother. The sun was shining, and he felt like he was walking on a cloud. He was baptized the following Sunday. Rod had already been baptized. Poofus began to ask Mother about being saved and baptized. She later learned that he began to dread being baptized because putting his head underwater caused him to choke violently.

Rod and Ronnie took a swimming lesson at Westmoreland Swimming Pool sponsored by the YMCA. They learned to hold their head underwater, float, tread water, dog-paddle, and finally to swim, all in one morning. Poofus never learned to do any of those water activities.

One movie night, it was raining hard nonstop for hours, so Mother decided not to take them. Poofus began to complain and beg her to take them anyway. *This going places in bad weather became a lifelong issue between them.* As usual, Mother gave in, drove them to the Roxy theater through almost flooded streets, told them she would pick them up when the movie was over, let them out in the drenching rain, and drove away. Soaking wet, they went in and watched the movie. After the cartoon and serial feature, they showed highlights of recent WWII battles, made an appeal to buy war bonds, and then began the main feature. It was about submarine battles with almost all underwater action. When it was over, Poofus and Ronnie rode home with Mother through flooded streets. Fortunately, it was only thirteen blocks to home. This was one time that Poofus and Ronnie did not act out the movie. They were waterlogged.

Every time Poofus would go to a movie, he would sit on the front row. Neither Mother nor Ronnie ever sat with him. They sat behind him about halfway back from the screen so they could watch him. Every time a scary or very loud scene came on, he would turn his head away from the screen, get down on his knees, and put his arms over his ears. He did that until Ronnie left home for college. Nobody knows when he stopped doing that.

After WWII, Uncle Sonny bought Chester Hallford's Service Station at 2210 Grant Street on the corner of Cumberland Avenue and was still half-owner of Stepp Brothers Grocery. He ran the station, and Daddy ran the grocery store while hiring family members to help. These included Aunt Lydia and nephews Buddy Bond, Paul Bond, and Lesley Bond. Sonny soon added an icehouse to his service station.

In August 1945, the Lee Roy Stepp family moved to 2208 Grant Street between the grocery store and Sonny's service station. Daddy bought the house from Chester Hallford. The Hallford family was always a part of their lives. Poofus was still sitting on the produce box, but not as often as before. He could easily be seen from their home when he did. They had a fenced-in backyard, and Poofus got his first puppy and named him Skippy. A month later, Uncle Sonny and Aunt Ruby moved to 3011 Avenue Q. The two Stepp families were now only six blocks apart.

Their former house, the duplex, was sold and moved off their lot at 2206 Grant Street. Ronnie kissed the back of the house as it was leaving their property.

Rod and Ronnie started third grade in early September 1945. Ms. Jewel Williamson was their teacher. They liked her very much. *Poofus still had never had a schoolteacher.* This is the year that Rod and Ronnie accelerated their development of reading skills. They brought many schoolbooks home to read, and Ronnie often read to Poofus, who also looked through all the books. In the summer, Ronnie checked out books from the Sam Houston grade school library. It was a good year of learning and playing softball and football in season with Rod and other boys. They played at home and at school at recess and often after school on the playgrounds. *Poofus could not join them in such play at this time*, but Roddy, Butch, and Ronnie still played army and cowboys with him.

Early in school year 1945–46, Ms. Hardeman took her eight-member square dance team, now in the third grade, to perform at Zundelowitz junior high school during the school day. Then she took them to perform at Iowa Park high school at night, and Mother took Poofus to see them. One night, they danced at the local United Services Organization (USO) for the military service personnel, and Poofus got to see them perform again. *He enjoyed the music and dancing very much, and he would be performing himself nine years later at a much larger venue.*

With WWII ending in October, all their uncles and cousins who fought in the war started coming home. Uncle Johna was the last to return, and the Ewing family got together to welcome him home. His weight had dropped from 180 pounds to 110 pounds while in Japanese work camps, but he had gained about 40 pounds during the months of getting home. Within a year, he was back to his normal weight. *By the grace of God, none of their relatives were lost in the war.*

Uncle Sonny and Uncle Louis began construction of a metal building on the former site of the duplex. It was designed to be a self-service laundry. As the end of construction neared, Rod and Ronnie delivered circulars door-to-door announcing the opening of the Westside Washateria at 2206 Grant Street. For some reason, Ronnie vividly remembers delivering the circulars in the Westover Hills subdivision, particularly to Lola Mae Knight Tompkins's home.

On December 17, 1945, Lee and Stella had their third son and named him David Loy. He was called David.

Christmas 1945 was better than the year before. Poofus got a book titled *Little Black Sambo*, a checker set, Crayola crayons, coloring books, clothes, and another toy pickup with side boards like Uncle John's. Ronnie got clothes including Levi's, two pairs of boxing gloves, a very used bicycle, and a football. Rod and Poofus were usually his boxing opponents. Daddy bought Mother a nice, used dining room set including a table with a pad, six chairs, a china closet, a buffet cabinet, and a long mirror to place above the buffet. Mother was proud of it the rest of her life.

Ronnie remembers going with Daddy to get the furniture at a house near Spudder Park, which was the home of the professional minor league baseball Spudders in the Class B Big State League. It was on a Sunday, and the Spudders were playing a game. He heard the loud roar of the crowd. It was his second time to see Spudder Park, but the first time to hear the fans there. Four years later, he would be playing there for the Greyhounds, and Poofus would be their batboy. Ronnie's first time to see Spudder Park was when Uncle Louis and Aunt Lydia took him to a circus in 1941.

At this time, life changed dramatically for the Lee Roy Stepp family. It changed especially for Mother and Poofus.

In March 1946, their family moved to a 160-acre farm just east of Hugo, Oklahoma. Daddy and Uncle Sonny had bought the property on January 1. Uncle John had moved back to a farm near Hugo about six months earlier. Daddy, Sonny, and John were born in Cooper, Texas, but moved from Cooper to Hugo in late December 1912. Their family made that move in a covered wagon. On that trip, Daddy had his eighth birthday on December 20. A few weeks later,

John had his tenth birthday on January 9, and Sonny had his fourth birthday on January 14. Ronnie thinks all three of them wanted to live close to one another on farms near where they had lived for ten years of their childhood.

Ronnie moved in with Rod's family until the end of school in late May. He was there for Butch's sixth birthday party on March 31. He missed Poofus's tenth birthday party on April 8, but he went to Rod's ninth birthday party on the same day. Then on May 1, Aunt Ruby gave him a birthday party. It was his ninth. She hosted three birthday parties in a period of four weeks and three days.

After school was out, Uncle Sonny and Aunt Ruby took Ronnie to his new home. He was looking forward to living on a farm, getting a horse, going squirrel hunting, fishing in the stock tank, etc., but he was going to miss all his family and friends back in Wichita Falls. Rod and his family visited with them two days and returned home. Their two families were now to be 210 miles apart.

Mother was now charged with caring for newborn David, special-needs Poofus, and Ronnie, with no help from the Ewing and Stepp families. Uncle John and Aunt Velma lived one mile from them, but they were always working daylight to after dark. Uncle John was still in the delivery business and took Poofus with him some. Aunt Velma had household chores, hogs to tend, and most time-consuming, she had to help her parents who lived just down the road. Her parents were in their early seventies and needed help with caring for two mules, four milk cows, six hogs, many chickens, a fruit garden, a large vegetable garden, and with canning some of the crops. Uncle John helped with the livestock.

Lee Roy's house had electricity, running water from a well with an electric pump in a small pump house, but no restroom. Ronnie does not remember being much help to Mother. *Thinking of those months now makes him appreciate Mother even more.*

The move's impact on Ronnie personally would not start dramatically until school started in September. He would have only one friend in school from the start. There would be no help or encouragement from older cousins, aunts, or uncles with his schoolwork. Poofus had not experienced the joy of having schoolmates.

Ronnie's favorite thing to do that summer was hunt squirrels with Uncle John's Winchester pump .22 rifle.[3] He also liked to sit on Aunt Velma's front porch and shoot at an empty Lucky Strike pack across the road. The red circle made a good target. The far side of the road had a four-foot bank with heavy woods behind it. The property was called Rose Hill. It was safe for target practice because of the clay bank, and he always made sure no motor vehicles or mule-drawn wagons were passing. He became a good shot with that rifle, and he ate squirrel often. Of course, Poofus could not shoot the rifle. But it would have been much more fun for Ronnie if Poofus had been born normal and could have gone squirrel hunting. Then when they treed a squirrel, the one who did not have the rifle could slowly walk around the tree's drip line to get the squirrel to move slowly around in the sight of the other who would be ready to shoot.

Daddy had bought a grocery store at the edge of Hugo. A three-room addition housed the previous owners. Daddy allowed them to live there until they found another house. They had a son, Tommy, one year younger than Ronnie, a daughter one year older, and another daughter in high school. Daddy allowed the older daughter to open the store each morning before he got there and to work part-time in the store as needed.

Daddy also bought a streetcar diner in the middle of town, which was a popular hamburger and hotdog business. The previous owner hired on to continue doing the cooking. These two businesses were doing well at that time.

Each week, Mother dropped Poofus and Ronnie off at one of the two movie theaters. The Durango Kid soon became Poofus's favorite western actor. Sunset Carson was his other favorite. Coming in third was Lash LaRue of bull whip fame. For some reason, they did not see any Gene Autry or Roy Rogers movies that summer. When they played cowboys, Poofus chose to be the Durango Kid, and he told Ronnie to be Sunset Carson, not Lash LaRue, because he did not want to get struck with a bull whip.

They joined Oak Grove Baptist Church just east of their farm on Oklahoma state Highway 70. The pastor's last name was McFarland. Early on, they went to Vacation Bible School. The church building had only one room, so children met in two or three corners by age groups. It was the same setup for Sunday school.

Often, Poofus would sit on the front porch of the house and watch long railroad trains go by parallel to the highway. *Poofus did not do much walking on the farm.* It might have been because he was afraid of snakes. Daddy taught Ronnie at this time to not fear snakes, to give them their distance, and to only kill the poisonous ones. Ronnie heeded that all his life.

Daddy soon bought a female bay horse named Fanny. Ronnie liked the horse but immediately started calling her Flicka.[4] Poofus would not have anything to do with her. What he enjoyed most was going to Aunt Velma's house with Mother.

While Ronnie was riding Flicka to Uncle John's with a blanket on her back but no saddle, she stepped on a partially exposed corrugated metal pipe culvert that crossed the dirt road, bucked high, and sent him flying. With some difficulty, he got her positioned in the roadside ditch so he could get back on her (he was always small for his age). Soon after that, Daddy bought a "brand-new" saddle. Ronnie often went horseback riding with Tommy. Poofus never wanted to get on the horse. It could have been his horse and saddle as well as Ronnie's.

Aunt Velma's father, Ivan Harrison Cody, hired a hay-baling crew each summer. Cousin Ivan "Sonny Boy" Stepp, son of Uncle John and Aunt Velma, worked on that crew, and he got his grandfather to hire Ronnie at fifty cents a day. Sonny Boy was eight years older than Poofus. He drove the tractor to mow the hay meadows and then to pull a sweeper to move the hay to the baling machine.

Ronnie's job was to grab a hay bale with a bale hook as it came out of the baler and to drag the bale to the stackers. That was not easy for him to do because the fifty- to sixty-pound bale of hay weighed almost as much as he did. He worked on six hay meadows and enjoyed all of them. The most difficult job was on Daddy's meadow because Ronnie also had to help stack the bales in the hot hay loft. *Poofus, though a year older, could not do that job.*

While working on the meadow of the property of a circus's winter quarters across the road from Daddy's store, Ronnie watched one of the baling crew grab a rattlesnake by the tail, swiftly swing it round and round over his head, and snap it like a whip, causing its head to pop off.[5] On Mr. Brown's meadow, which was about one mile due south of Daddy's house, a large tomato patch was near the meadow. During the working day, Ronnie picked several tomatoes, dusted them off, salted them, and ate them. Sonny Boy told him about the tomato patch the day before, so Ronnie took a saltshaker in a pocket of his bib overalls. Thankfully, Poofus did not know what he was missing.

One day, Mr. Ivan Cody took Ronnie with him to town in his wagon pulled by his two mules. He did not have a motor vehicle. It was five and a half miles from his house to town. They talked most of the time while going and coming. Mr. Cody shopped for groceries and livestock feed while Ronnie looked around, and then they went back to the Cody house. It took about six hours. Ronnie always enjoyed visiting with him.

Norita Cody, niece of Aunt Velma, was Ronnie's first girlfriend. They had first met and played several times when she visited Uncle John and Aunt Velma in Wichita Falls two and three years earlier. They got to play together some that summer. One day they played with four or five other kids in the Rose Hill at the old Colonel Robert McDonald Jones family cemetery.

But fortunately for Mother, Poofus, Ronnie, and David, their short stay in Hugo ended in mid-August 1946.

Daddy discovered that the family living temporarily in his house attached to his grocery store were stealing money from the store cash register and groceries. They also owed Daddy several months of rent that they had agreed to pay. When the man told Daddy that his family was going to stay until evicted, Daddy decided that he would not evict them because of the children. He began to open, operate, and close the store himself.

A few days later, Daddy was informed by the county clerk that the streetcar diner property had some legal issues that had just been discovered and that they must be corrected soon. After getting more details and learning how much it might cost to get everything in order, Daddy decided to sell out and go back to Wichita Falls.

Daddy sold the two businesses for less than he paid for them. He and Sonny sold the 160 acres, house, and barn for about what they paid for them. Daddy sold the horse and saddle, and he hired a cattle truck driver to move his furniture and household items back to Wichita Falls. They followed the truck in Daddy's 1939 Chevrolet sedan. Daddy sold the car immediately after the trip to give them some money to live on.

Moving back at that time in Poofus's life would change his future for the better exponentially. If the move to Oklahoma had been good for Daddy financially, it would not have been as good for Mother, Poofus, Ronnie, and David.

Their return to Wichita Falls at that time would also be fortunate for Rod, because in Ronnie's short absence, Rod had gotten in bad trouble with his mother. He had played *marbles for keeps* with four older boys (at least one was five years older) in the neighborhood. Aunt Ruby had told Rod that he was not to play marbles for keeps. When he got home with a large bag full of marbles, Aunt Ruby asked him how he came by them. When Rod told her that he had played marbles for keeps with Bobby Howard and three other boys, she told him to take them back right then and give them back their marbles. When Rod tried to give them back, Bobby said he could not take them because Rod had won them "fair and square." The other boys did the same. Rod does not remember what he did with the marbles, but Aunt Ruby never saw them again. After that, Rod never played marbles for keeps. A few years later, Bobby was one of the best baseball players in high school and then played professionally and made it to class AAA. That used bicycle Ronnie got for Christmas 1945 was bought from Bobby.

For two months, they lived with Uncle Louis and Aunt Lydia. They had a daughter, Mona Gayle, who was soon to be six years old. Poofus and Ronnie enjoyed living with them. Mona taught Ronnie to play *ball and jacks*. Poofus was not able to join them in that game. But he did play with them when Mona was in charge as they *played house*. She bossed them around and made them enjoy it. The six Stepp boys had no sisters and did not know about the manipulative skills of girls at that time. Susie Bond, Dora Bond's daughter, often joined Mona in "bossing the Stepp boys around."

Mother now had her strong family and church support again, and her daily mothering tasks did not require all her time. But she was still concerned about Poofus not being educated in public schools.

School year 1946–47 began for Rod and Ronnie, but Poofus was still not able to attend school. Ms. Esther Berry, who was like a female General Dwight D. Eisenhower to Ronnie in a positive sense, was still their principal. They began their first year with different teachers for each subject. Ms. Carrye Smith[6] taught math, Ms. Eura Mae Haggard taught geography and history, Ms. Edith Denton taught English and literature, Ms. Mary Hindman taught reading, writing, and spelling. Ms. Burt taught art and Spanish and Ms. Fernetta Foley taught music. Wow. Did they ever have a lot to learn? And they thrived on it. Also, they had more fun in recess playing softball and football in season. Poofus was missing so much, and Rod and Ronnie wished he could do more things with them.

In English class, Ms. Denton required them to memorize and quote selected poems. She said that poems they memorized at their age would never be forgotten. She was right. Ronnie memorized and quoted "Trees" by Joyce Kilmer and "Stopping by Woods on a Snowy Evening" by Robert Frost and still quotes them to this day. The primary reason that he can still recite them is that he quotes them every four or five years. Ms. Denton knew that would be the case for many of her students. At the time of rewriting this chapter, the USA is still experiencing closures of churches because of Covid-19. Ronnie started a family Bible study on Sundays with eight adults attending. They are using the same memorization of scripture technique that Ms. Denton taught Ronnie in the 1940s for memorizing poems.

But at this time, a divine appointment occurred in the lives of Mother, Poofus, and his only public schoolteacher.

Mother had parked downtown to go into a store to make a quick purchase. She left Poofus in the car. A woman noticed him, and seeing he had no hands, she went closer to him and saw that he had no feet. She spoke to him and got some response. Having worked with children as a special education teacher for many years, she could understand him better than most. After they talked for a few minutes, Mother returned and introduced herself and Poofus to Mrs. Thelma Williams. Mrs. Williams told Mother that Poofus had a bright mind and should be in school and that she currently was teaching a special education class at Austin grade school. Mother said she wanted to get him in that class as soon as possible.

Mother had been praying for years that God would make provisions for Poofus to go to school. Mrs. Williams told Mother to bring him to Austin grade school the next day and the principal would be notified that Shelby and Mother were coming. Mother told her that she already knew the principal, Mr. Woodward, because he had lived next door to her for six years.

Poofus started public school education in early September 1946.

The next day, Poofus was enrolled in the special education class at Austin grade school. *He now had his first schoolteacher.* He had missed the first two weeks of school year 1946–47, but he made up for it and more. Of course, God had made the connection, and both lives were blessed for many years. Mrs. Williams would be an unbelievable teacher for Poofus, and Poofus would be a remarkable student for Mrs. Williams. She was all that Mother had been praying for to help Poofus in his schooling and ability to live a good, meaningful, and rewarding life.

Mrs. Williams had worked with handicapped children since 1937, but Poofus would give her some new challenges and many rewarding years of achievement. She received a bachelor of arts degree from Daniel Baker College in Brownwood, Texas, and had done postgraduate work at the University of Texas and Texas Christian University.

Mrs. Williams quickly realized that Poofus had a sharp mind and was able to read and spell already at first grade level. He learned rapidly, and she kept challenging him and giving him opportunities to achieve more.

In late October 1946, Daddy bought a house at 2608 Grant Street from Mr. Cage and his family moved in. It had a tall fence in the backyard, so Poofus got a very athletic black and brown terrier that he named Bill. That dog could really run and jump. Poofus had a lot of fun running with Bill in the backyard.

Daddy was soon back in the grocery business at 2206 Grant Street, and his financial situation improved steadily. One Sunday in late 1946, he took Ronnie downtown to a drugstore with a soda fountain and ordered two ham and cheese sandwiches and two milkshakes. Then they went to the Strand Theater nearby and saw the movie *The Yearling*. Ronnie does not remember what the occasion was, but he surely enjoyed it. In the grocery business, Daddy always worked Monday through Saturday from 7:00 a.m. to 9:00 p.m. In all of Ronnie's years of playing baseball and softball, his daddy only came to two games, but Ronnie did not blame him because he was always working.

For the first time by themselves, Rod and Ronnie rode a city bus to downtown. They went to a movie theater and saw Wallace Beery and Margaret O'Brien in *Bad Bascomb*. It was about an outlaw who joins a Mormon wagon train to hide out after a failed bank robbery. Bascomb undergoes a reformation during his interactions with a young girl who becomes attached to him. It was a good story, and it had a good ending. Their visit downtown would have had a better ending if they had taken Poofus with them. Mother was cautious about letting him go anywhere without her.

For Christmas 1946, Poofus got his first tricycle. It was new with bright red and white paint. *He soon was riding frequently two blocks to Aunt Ruby's house.* From a distance, he looked like a normal boy riding his tricycle. Ronnie got a football uniform and a new Nocona baseball glove. One-year-old David got a tin spinning top and a big red, white, and blue ball. As usual, they all got some clothes and books.

Bill, Poofus's dog, jumped over their five-foot fence, ate some rat poison in Ray's Hatchery feed storage building nearby, and died a painful death. Mother soon got Poofus another dog, a six-month-old German shepherd. Poofus named him Rusty and said he was going to grow up to be like Rin-Tin-Tin. Five months later someone left a gate open, and Rusty was hit by a car on Grant Street and was killed instantly. Poofus did not get another dog for several years.

AN INCREDIBLE BOY AND A REMARKABLE MAN

At the end of school year 1946–47, *Poofus completed first and second grade requirements with high grades! He made two grades in his first year*! Rod and Ronnie also made high grades and were promoted to fifth grade.

Rod and Ronnie began to play softball after school on the Sam Houston ball field. They usually had eight or nine players, and they played what was called scrub. They had three players batting and the others at the positions of pitcher, first baseman, shortstop, left fielder, and right fielder. When a batter made an out or was tagged out running the bases, he would become the right fielder. The other fielders would always rotate pitcher to hitter, first baseman to pitcher, shortstop to first baseman, left fielder to shortstop, and right fielder to left fielder. If all three hitters ended up being on base with no one to bat, the runner on third base would be declared "out" and would become the right fielder, and the rotation of fielders would be made. They had no catcher, and the umpiring was done collectively by all players. That umpiring activity taught them how to "negotiate" and be fair. They enjoyed playing "scrub ball" for five or six years. Poofus was not able to play these games with them because of the longer distances to throw and larger areas to cover in the field.

Early in the summer of 1947, Poofus's crossed eyes had begun giving him trouble as his reading time had rapidly increased. Mother asked their family doctor for a referral to an eye surgeon who could do the corrective eye surgery. The doctor told her he would get right back to her. Ronnie does not know the details of what took place, but a local businessman who had heard about Poofus needing eye surgery got involved. Very soon, Poofus, Mother, and the businessman[7] went by rail to Saint Louis, Missouri, and successful surgery was performed.

Ronnie's practice of reading books each summer continued. He checked a book out of the school library, and after reading it, he became a New York Yankee fan. The title of the book was *Pride of the Yankees*. Mother, Poofus, and Ronnie had seen the movie of the same title the year before.

It was the story of Lou Gehrig, the first baseman of the Yankees from 1923–1939. He was nicknamed "The Iron Horse" because of his 2,130 consecutive games played, which was the major league record for many decades. Ronnie remembered that record all his life although it was broken by Cal Ripken fifty-six years later. Cal was another fine gentleman in Major League Baseball. Ronnie still considers Lou Gehrig to be the greatest man and ballplayer of all time.

Most of the other books Ronnie read that school year and summer were biographies of Daniel Boone and Davy Crockett, a history of Texas, and stories about boys and their dogs and horses written by Thomas C. Hinkle. He read some of them to Poofus

They did not go to movies as often now. There ceased to be a movie night. But they did enjoy Tarzan movies with Johnny Weissmuller and Abbott and Costello movies, but they did not reenact them when they got home as before. However, during the *Abbott and Costello Meet Frankenstein* movie, Poofus got scared and went down on the floor many times to avoid seeing Frankenstein.

Cousin Charles Bond took Rod and Ronnie to the Cedar Park swimming pool across from Hardin College several times that summer. Although the pool had no shade, the water was cooler than that at the Westmoreland Swimming Pool where they usually went to swim.

Ronnie began to read the sports section of the *Wichita Falls Daily Times* and *Wichita Falls Record News*. He followed the games of the Wichita Falls Spudders professional baseball team and the New York Yankees. His favorite active Yankee was Joe Dimaggio. Poofus and Ronnie began to listen to the Spudders games on Daddy's radio. Al "Red" McCarty was the favorite hitter of Poofus. His favorite pitcher was Sid Peterson. McCarty and Peterson played all six years that they followed the team. Ronnie got to go to one game with a friend whose dad took them, but Mother would not let Poofus go because he would have to ride in the bed of the pickup with Ronnie.

In August 1947, Daddy bought the house at 3105 York Street from Mr. Hyde whose son Teddy was the same age as Poofus. For many years before, it was the only house in the block bounded by York Street, Garfield Road, Avenue Q, and Santa Fe Road. They now lived only two blocks from Uncle Sonny's house. For Poofus and Ronnie, it became the favorite house of their childhood. They played a lot of football and baseball in the front yard and backyard, which were all grass.

In that home, their family settled into a daily routine. They would all get up by 6:00 a.m. and get ready for the day. Mother would cook breakfast, and they would eat as a family, but Mother never sat down at the table even though there was room. While they were eating, Daddy liked to kid around with his sons, but Shelby was too intent on eating, and David was too young to pester, so Ronnie became the primary target. Within four years, he would begin doing the same with David. Poofus would feed himself and did not have time to talk. Daddy would finish first and go to his grocery store. He would not come home from work until after 9:00 p.m. Poofus and Ronnie went to school, came home to play, ate a family meal without Daddy, and played again until bedtime. Most of what they learned at home about life, they learned from Mother.

What they learned at home about life was much the same as what they learned at school about life, which was much the same as what they learned at church about life, which was much the same as what they learned in the neighborhood about life, which was much the same about what they learned about life in the books they read, in the movies they saw, and in the radio shows they heard. In the 1990s, Ronnie started telling Rod, Jim B., Jim P., and Bill McFall when they all got together that their generation had it better than any before or after them. They always agreed with him. Ronnie also shared that same thought with Poofus. With all his handicaps, Poofus was blessed in this most important spiritual aspect of life. In less than a year, he would make the most important decision of his life.

Most nights, ten or twelve boys and girls in their neighborhood would gather in the 3100 block of Avenue Q and play hide-and-seek and kick the can, etc. They would play until their mothers called them home. Poofus never showed any interest in playing those games at night. He enjoyed playing his records and listening to the radio and reading books.

School year 1947–48, Poofus's spiritual, school, and social life continued to broaden. He began to converse more frequently with his classmates and students from other classes. They had difficulty understanding his speech, and he struggled to understand his classmates that had cerebral palsy. But friendships at church and school began to blossom. He improved his reading skills and handwriting and made high grades in all subjects. He went to church every Sunday morning and night, and he also went every Wednesday night.

But at the age of eleven, Poofus committed his first improper act. While sitting on the curb with four-year-old Jim Stepp in front of Aunt Ruby's house, he told Jim to holler "you h——y butt" at motorists as they drove by. Most cars had no air conditioner, and drivers usually had their windows down. Poofus and Jim did this repeatedly until a motorist stopped, and a man got out and took Jim by the hand to the front door of his house and knocked. Aunt Ruby came to the door, and the man told her what had happened. Aunt Ruby apologized, thanked the man, and told him that she would punish Jim right then. When she began to whip Jim, Poofus did not confess that he caused Jim to do it. *That was two wrongs for Poofus.* Ronnie does not know if Mother or Aunt Ruby ever knew what Poofus had done. *This event was before he made his profession of faith in Christ as his Savior and Lord.*

Christmas 1947, a tradition began for the six Stepp boys. Rod, Butch, and Jim would get up early and open their gifts. Then they would run two blocks to the other Stepp house and wake them up and watch them open their gifts. Usually, they would bring their favorite gift. They always had good gifts and good times at Christmas. Some years, Ronnie is not sure about certain gifts, but they included clothes, books, sports equipment, bicycles, table games, records, watches, billfolds, Bibles, and toys. Rod and Ronnie ceased participation in 1960 because they each married and left Wichita Falls.

School year 1947–48, Rod and Ronnie were in fifth grade and had mostly the same teachers as in the fourth grade. Ms. Rebecca Craig was their new art, music, and Spanish teacher. Ms. Haggard taught Texas history, and they each got a free paperback book from the Magnolia Mobil Oil Company. The title was *Texas History Movies Book*. It had nothing to do with movies, but it told the story of the history of Texas from European exploration to American statehood in comic strip form. Ronnie still has his copy, but it is missing the front cover and several of the early pages. He bought a later edition in 2000 for his grandchildren. In early 2020, he bought another copy to educate his great-grandchildren. In English class, Ms. Denton encouraged the students to buy books through the school. Ronnie bought *Johnny Tremain*, which was a good historical fiction book. Poofus also read it and discussed it with Ronnie. Same as last year, she required memorizing and reciting selected poems. Ronnie memorized and recited "Daffodils" or "I Wandered Lonely as a Cloud" by William Wordsworth and "Sea Fever" by John Masefield. He is still grateful to Ms. Denton for encouraging memorization of poems.

Ms. Smith continued to make learning mathematics a lot of fun. And she taught her students much more than math. On the front wall above the blackboard, she displayed colorful cards with character-building statements. Ronnie's two favorites were:

> *"I complained because I had no shoes until I met a man who had no feet"* and *"Do the best you can with what you have."* (The second statement was similar to what Pastor Huff[8] said at the beginning of each day of Vacation Bible School: *"I will do the best I can, with what I have, where I am today."*) Of course, both statements reminded Ronnie of Poofus, and throughout his life, Poofus reminded Ronnie of those two quotations.

Ms. Smith also supervised the boys' softball team when they practiced and played other schools. As an indicator of her success with them, though they missed winning the YMCA grade school city championship game in the sixth grade by one run on a controversial call by an umpire, they were good sports and did not complain. But more of a tribute to her came six years later, when the HHBC church softball team was the undefeated champion of the YMCA Senior Youth League. Their record for the season was seventeen wins and no losses. At the awards banquet at Floral Heights Methodist Church, as captain of the team, Ronnie not only went forward to receive the team championship trophy, but he was called forward again to receive the team sportsmanship trophy. *Eight of the nine starters of that team had been taught by Ms. Smith. And Poofus was the batboy for that team.*

One day after school, Ronnie was walking to a Royal Ambassadors[9] meeting at HHBC across the street from Sam Houston. As he walked on the grass lawn of the church, he was knocked down flat on his face from behind with somebody sitting on his back and pounding on both sides of his head. Suddenly, the person pulled off Ronnie, and when he got up, Jimmy Pitts was hitting Joe Brooks Cleveland and telling him never to bother Ronnie again. Joe was the same size as Jimmy and much bigger than Ronnie. When Poofus was told what had happened, he said that Jim Pitts was his hero.

The next day in school, Ms. Berry called Jimmy, Joe, and Ronnie to her office and questioned them about what had happened in the fight yesterday. Jimmy told her the truth about what he saw and did. Ronnie told her the truth about the little he saw and did. Ronnie does not remember what Joe said. Ms. Berry then talked to each of them privately. She told Ronnie that he had done nothing wrong and dismissed him. Jimmy told Ronnie later that she told him that he had done right, but that he must avoid fighting if possible. Jimmy and Ronnie did not know how she punished Joe, but knowing her policy about fighting, they were confident that she admonished him, advised him not to start fights, and gave him a whipping. Ronnie never did know why Joe did not like him.

For the first time, Rod and Ronnie rode their bicycles from home to downtown. They looked at Mickey Mouse watches at Zales Jewelers and browsed at Kress's, McCrory's, Woolworth's, and Huffhines Sporting Goods. They do not remember ever riding their bicycles downtown again.

In April 1948, Poofus, who had just turned twelve, was visiting Aunt Ruby in her home when the following occurred, in his own words:

> *"I accepted Christ as my personal Savior one day in the Spring of 1948 at the age of twelve. I was baptized a few days later, on Easter Sunday in the evening service. There were two people most influ-*

ential in my conversion… Mother and Aunt Ruby. I learned about Jesus while listening to Mother read the Bible to me at home and her Bible storytelling in Sunday school class. The true meaning of Calvary came to me one day while visiting Aunt Ruby. I was looking through an illustrated Bible and came across a picture of Jesus hanging on a cross. I asked Aunt Ruby what Jesus had done to deserve such a terrible punishment. She said that sin had become a barrier between God and man and that Jesus had so much love for us that he was willing to die on the cross and shed his blood for the remission of our sins. I was baptized in the Easter Sunday evening service, and Pastor Huff held a folded handkerchief over my mouth and nose while my head was underwater."

At the end of school year 1947–48, *Poofus completed third and fourth grade requirements! He had made four grades in his first two years in school! Rod and Ronnie thought he would catch up with them by the end of the next school year.* All three of them made high grades. Ronnie's readings continued to be biographies, histories, and stories of boys and dogs and horses. Some of the books were *Kit Carson, Buffalo Bill,* and *Black Beauty*. Poofus read all or parts of some of them too.

The summer of 1948 was the first year that Rod and Ronnie played in the YMCA Kid Baseball program. They played for the Panthers in the Midget League (ages eleven to twelve). Ronnie was pitcher, Rod played left field, Jim Booher played right field, and Jimmy Pitts played shortstop. The day before their first game, Rod and Ronnie went to Huffhines Sporting Goods to buy a bat. The owner, Mr. Austin Huffhines, helped them select a bat. He asked them what team they played for. When he was told, he said, "You are playing the Wildcats tomorrow, which is my son's team. If you win the game, come in and see me, and I will give you any bat you choose." It was not a bet. They had nothing to lose. All they had to do to get it was to win the game.

The next day, Rod, Ronnie, Jim B., Charles Wesson, and several others walked two miles to Hamilton Park. They played the Wildcats and beat them in the last inning by a score of 8 to 7. English Pharmacy was their team sponsor, and Mr. English had told them to come for a free fountain drink after each game they won. They went immediately after their first win, and most got milkshakes. The next day, Rod and Ronnie went to see Mr. Huffhines and picked out a purple Ty Cobb bat. He was so gracious to do that. It became their team's favorite bat.

In 1951, Travis Huffhines and Jack Roberts from that Wildcat team joined Ronnie and Jimmy on the Broncos team. Over the years, Rod and Ronnie bought many items from Mr. Huffhines's stores. The Panthers won their first ten games (they went to English Pharmacy for milkshakes after each game) and ended the season with a record of fourteen wins and two losses, and they finished in third place in the league. Mother brought Poofus to most of the games.

At home in his backyard, Ronnie began to play more serious football and baseball with Poofus simulating real games. In their imaginary high school football and baseball games, Poofus's team was the Vega Greyhounds and Ronnie's was the Northrop Broncos. In college games, Poofus's team was the Sam Houston Indians, and Ronnie's was the Jefferson Broncos. When playing with Poofus, Ronnie would play at slower speeds in both sports, and in baseball, he would bat left-handed instead of his natural right-handed and throw much easier.

At other times, Rod and a few other boys often played with Poofus and Ronnie. They all did what they could to enable Poofus to compete with them and be on the winning team half of the time. Poofus and Ronnie also played football *on the road*.[10] In his memorabilia, Ronnie has a small envelope with a bridal shower invitation for August 30, 1948, in it. On the envelope in pencil is a written note to Mother saying, "Me and Poofus are over at Ruby's playing football. Ronald."

Poofus and Ronnie continued to follow the Spudders on the radio and in the newspaper, and Ronnie also followed the Yankees and Dimaggio. Rod and Poofus began to keep up with their favorite teams in Major League Baseball. They both became fans of the Cleveland Indians in the American League and the Brooklyn Dodgers in the National League. Ronnie favored the Saint Louis Cardinals in the National League because of Stan Musial, but he did not follow them as he did the Yankees. This made for verbal battles between Ronnie pulling for the Yankees and Poofus and Rod backing their two teams. This battle became strong from 1948 to 1958. It was two against one, but Ronnie's team beat their teams nearly every year. Poofus started liking Rod more and Ronnie less in some areas of life.

Like the year before, Ronnie got to go to one Spudder baseball game with his friend, and they saw Spudder left fielder, D. C. "Pud" Miller, hit three homeruns. Ronnie remembers the exact date of that night game because they announced midgame that Babe Ruth had just died. It was August 16, 1948. When Ronnie got home, he told Poofus that Babe Ruth died. It made Poofus sad. Like most kids, he liked *the Babe* even though he was a Yankee.

From this point on Poofus will be called "Shelby." Some of the oldest family members continued to call him Poofus, but Ronnie joined the majority of friends and family who began to call him Shelby. It is meaningful to me that just as Saul of Tarsus, a harsh persecutor of Christians, became Paul of Antioch after his conversion experience on the road to Damascus, Poofus became Shelby shortly after his conversion experience. He began a long life of being a loyal disciple of Jesus Christ.

School year 1948–1949, Shelby's third year under Mrs. Williams, she took him to a speech class on the North Texas State Teachers College campus in Denton, Texas. After an all-day class of learning the basics of improving speech, they came back and began to spend multiple hours each week training in breath control with Shelby using his diaphragm and speaking simple words formed from his vocal cords. Additionally, Mrs. Williams taught him to use his throat muscles to complement his vocal cords. His speech began to noticeably improve.

One week before Christmas at Austin grade school, Shelby played a piano concert of Christmas carols in the cafeteria for the students, cafeteria workers, and a newspaper photographer. He played only the simple melodies and hit a few wrong notes, but his audience was delighted. He told them that he wanted someday to lead his own music band.

After school on weekdays, Ronnie occasionally worked in Daddy's grocery store. He waited on cash and credit customers at checkout. For credit customers, he had to print or write cursive in the customers record book with carbon copy every item and price. Most credit customers paid their balance each month. He also swept the floor and dusted the items on shelves. On Saturdays, he worked longer hours. Shelby did not work in the grocery store until much later.

Rod and Ronnie continued with high grades in the sixth grade. Their teachers were the same as the year before except Ms. Bettye Birk became their art and Spanish teacher. They began to take violin lessons at school, and they were starters on the softball and touch football teams. Mr. Mike Locascio was their violin teacher and played in the Wichita Falls Symphony Orchestra. The students often got him to play "Flight of the Bumblebee" and "Goofus." He played them fast and professionally. Rod and Ronnie were impressed that he was also a boxer.

In English class, Ms. Denton continued to assign poems for memorization and recitation. Ronnie memorized and recited the required lines of "Rime of the Ancient Mariner" by Samuel Taylor Coleridge and all of "A Psalm of Life" by Henry Wadsworth Longfellow. He quoted the latter several times each year. He recited it in full during a presentation at church in 1997. He bought a book, *Bat Boy of the Giants*, based on a true story. Shelby probably read it since he had become a batboy. If the title had been *Bat Boy of the Dodgers*, he certainly would have read it.

The six Stepp boys observed their ritual early Christmas Day 1948. Shelby got a record player. His favorite recording artists were Gene Autry, Tex Ritter, and Red Foley. He played his records often. It was amazing to see him open the lid of his record player, pick up a forty-five-rpm or seventy-eight-rpm record, place the hole in the center of the record on the spindle of the turntable, drop the record onto the turntable, lift the tone arm and position it over the first track of the record, and lower the tone arm until the stylus contacted the record surface. He could not replace the stylus or cartridge. He did this often for the next three decades of his life using two record players. Shelby was becoming a happier boy each year.

Ronnie got a baseball table game that Shelby, Rod, Butch, and others enjoyed playing. It had a ball diamond to set on a table. At home plate was a metal spinner shaped like an arrow. The player at bat would select a major league player's template to place around the spinner. Templates were available for many former star players like Babe Ruth and Ty Cobb and active players like Stan Musial and Ted Williams. The spinner would be spun, the point would stop over "single," "fly out," "strikeout," etc. on the template. The size of each sector on the template was based on that player's lifetime major league batting statistics. For example, Babe Ruth's "home run" sector was the largest of all. Shelby's team of Dodgers and Indians sometimes beat Ronnie's team of Yankees. A paper pad of scoreboard format sheets was provided.

* * * * *

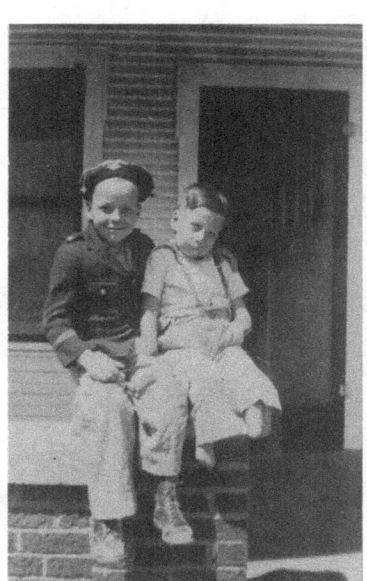

Shelby and Ron at 2804 Avenue L in 1944 about the time he learned to walk in the room behind him

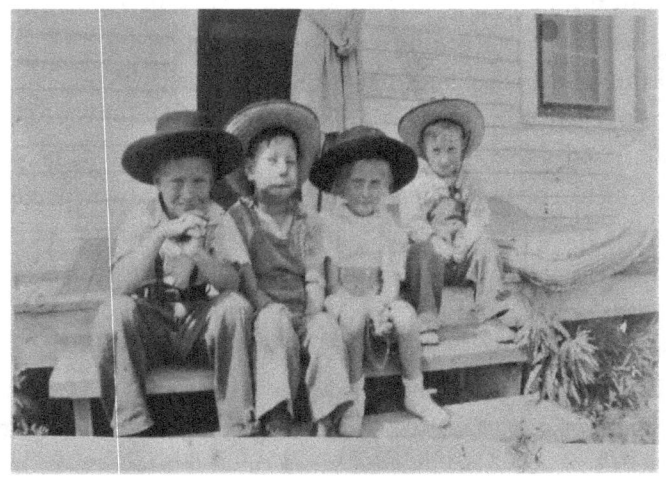

Butch, Shelby, Mona Watkins, and Jim at the
Stepp farm near Hugo, Ok in 1946

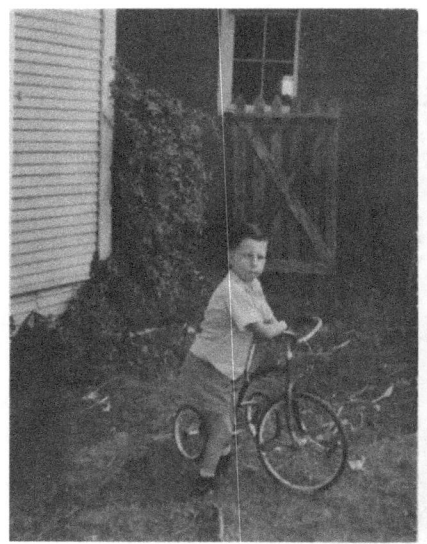 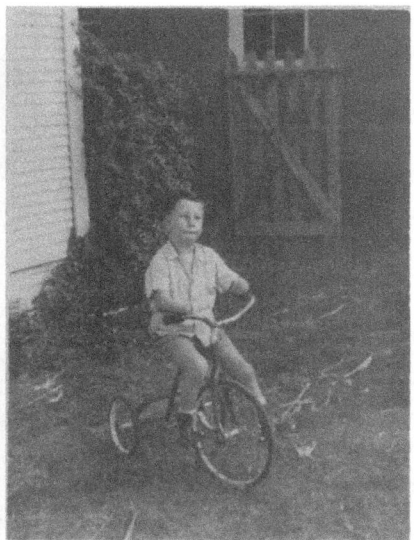

Shelby at 2608 Grant Street in 1947

AN INCREDIBLE BOY AND A REMARKABLE MAN

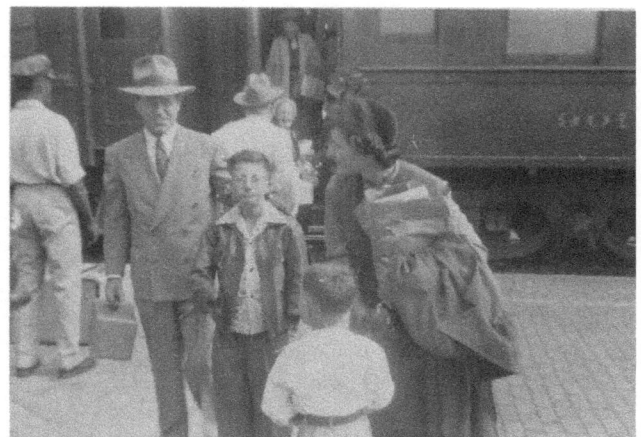

Frank Wood, Shelby, David, and Mother returning from Saint Louis after Shelby's crossed eyes were surgically corrected in 1948.

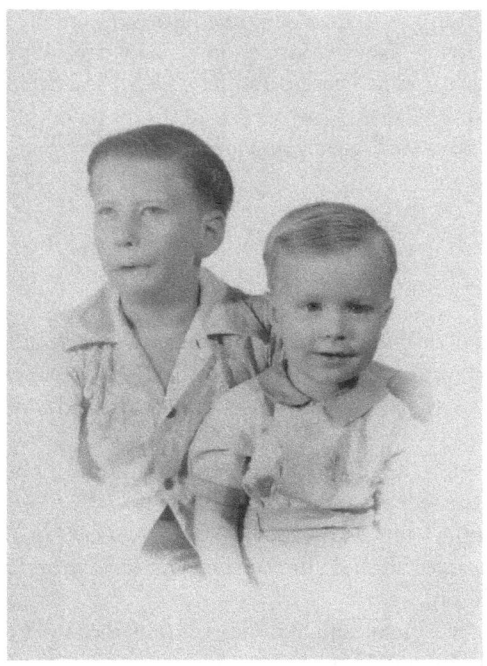

Shelby and David in September 1948 (age 12 yrs 5mos and 2 yrs 9 mos)

RONALD STEPP

---

[1] Passed by Mrs. L. R. Stepp PFC Willie Ewing

> Dear Ronnie, Poofus, Rodie, and Butch,
>
> I am writing to you because I have never answered your letters. The censor will probably think you are all in one family, but that is the only way I could think to write to you all. Ronnie you and Rodie will probably start to school this year. That means you are six.
>
> I hope you make good grades the first grade when I get home I will help you with your lessons. This is your old uncle. writing to you. Well, I mean your young uncle writing to you from away over the pool. Maybe some time I will let Johna loose from prison and we will come home together. Ruby that means mother has sons in the Army, Navy, Marines now. Son probably went in as a ensign and Johna is a 1st LT and me a first class private but in the best service. May God bless you all. Stella this is to you too.
>
> Your Uncle and Bro.
> Pfc Willie Ewing

[2] Most streets and neighborhoods in Wichita Falls were safe for children to walk and play in until the 1960s. Motorists slowed down when children were in or near the street, and child abusers, molesters, and kidnappers were very uncommon.

[3] A Winchester Pump .22 rifle model 62. In 1950, Ronnie bought a Winchester Pump .22 rifle model 62A and still has it.

[4] Poofus and Ronnie had seen the movie *My Friend Flicka* in 1944.

[5] In 1965, Ronnie saw a man do the same to a rattlesnake on Kemp Boulevard in Wichita Falls, Texas.

[6] Ms. Smith taught Mother and Ronnie's future father-in-law at Sam Houston grade school twenty-four years earlier.

[7] Ronnie is almost sure it was Frank Wood. If you know the identity of this businessman, please contact Ronald L Stepp at (713) 299-0348 or e-mail ronstepp37@yahoo.com.

8 Poofus, Rod, and Ronnie were baptized by Pastor A. C. Huff at Highland Heights Baptist Church in Wichita Falls, Texas.

9 Royal Ambassadors (RAs) is a Southern Baptist missions organization for boys in grades 1–6 that helps them develop a biblical worldview with an emphasis on missions learning and missions doing. RAs utilizes activities that are designed to help boys learn about missions and get them personally involved in practical mission experiences while having fun.

10 League and conference team sporting events are usually played at a team's field or stadium (home) or at the opponent's field or stadium (on the road).

CHAPTER 3

Early Teen Years: Thirteen to Fifteen (1949–51)

That same school year 1948–49, Shelby demonstrated his skill in printing and writing legibly, cutting with scissors (try that with your two fists), throwing darts, catching balls, helping dress himself, and many other things most his age do easily, but it was difficult for him.

Mrs. Williams said that he had spread out a sweater tied around his neck one day, and flapping his short arms, he cried out, "I am Superman." All his classmates and fellow students at Austin and classmates at Sunday school picked up on that nickname for him for a while.

She also said at this time, "Teaching a boy with such a quick and agile mind is a pleasure. When in competition with other fifth graders, he comes out with the best of them." But it did take Shelby longer to complete tests because he wrote and printed slowly.

Uncle Sonny built a concrete block building at the southwest corner of Grant Street and York Street. It was Stepp's Humble Service Station with two gasoline pumps and a bay with a hydraulic lift for lubricating and washing automobiles. He opened in mid-1949. The address was 2600 Grant Street.

One afternoon, Joe Cleveland picked a fight with Jerry Box on a vacant lot one block west of Jerry's house on Avenue Q. Rod and

AN INCREDIBLE BOY AND A REMARKABLE MAN

Ronnie watched and hoped that Jerry would win the fight. They were about the same size, but Jerry was not a fighter. Joe was getting the best of Jerry when Uncle Harry "Boydie" came along and took care of Joe and sent him home. (In school year 1952–1953, Joe failed the tenth grade in high school. He repeated the tenth grade, but he did not attend school after that. In the late 1950s, Joe got in a fight with an airman from Sheppard Air Force Base and was stabbed in the buttocks. That is all Ronnie knows about Joe. He should have taken to heart the advice that Ms. Berry gave him in her office back in 1948.)

Soon after that fight, Jerry Box, Douglas Box, and Ronnie were playing in the backyard of a house under construction next door to the Box's house. The house was being constructed with concrete blocks, and it had two unfinished walls that were two and three feet high. They were running and jumping over the short walls. Douglas was outjumping the others. A large boy the same age as Douglas who lived four blocks away in the Crockett school district walked up and began to say negative things to Douglas. His name was Hugh Moore, and he was taller and more muscular than Douglas.

About the time that Hugh was forcing a fight on Douglas, Jim Booher walked up from his house across the street and told Hugh to move on. Hugh threw one punch at Jim, and Jim threw the rest. Hugh went home, and the others told Jim how much they appreciated his help. Shelby was watching from his backyard and later told Ronnie that he was proud of Jim and that Jim was his hero. Both of Shelby's heroes were named Jim at this point. Ronnie never saw Hugh in the neighborhood after that day. Shelby, Rod, and Ronnie always thought Jim Booher was the best all-around boy and man their age that they ever knew.

When the Ewing family got together during his teen years, Shelby enjoyed "cutting up" (a positive activity) with cousin Jerry Ewing more than anyone. Jerry was four years older than Shelby and had one leg crippled by polio. Shelby enjoyed visiting everyone at those family events. Uncle Ike lived too far away to come to Wichita Falls during that period.

Wichita Falls public school superintendent Mr. Joe B. McNeil allowed students to go barefoot to school during hot weather. Rod and Ronnie did go barefoot, but Shelby did not. A new boy had come to Sam Houston for this school year and was in the sixth grade. Ronnie only saw him during recess. Physically he was tall with a better build than most boys in the sixth grade, but more importantly to Ronnie, he was Charley and Johnny Deal's brother. Ronnie was excited about him playing on the school softball and football teams, but he did not play either sport well. That was a big disappointment to Ronnie, and it puzzled him.

After school, Shelby often played with Jim S., Butch, David, and Joe Hallford. Usually, they played with toy cars and trucks on roads that they made in the shade of a chinaberry tree in Aunt Ruby's backyard. They also played cowboys and outlaws and army at war.

Near the end of school year 1948–1949, three of Ronnie's classmates were "cutting up" (a negative activity) in Spanish class. Ms. Birk would say a sentence in Spanish, and the class would repeat the sentence in unison. But each time for three or four sentences in a row, you could hear boy voices speaking gibberish and then giggling. *Ronnie recognized the voice of the culprits.* Ms. Birk stopped the learning exercise and asked the boys who were misbehaving to stand up. Nobody stood. Ms. Birk sent a student to get Ms. Berry. When Ms. Berry came, it was obvious that Ms. Birk was telling her what had happened. Ms. Berry then expressed her disappointment in the class and said that the class would have to stay after school.

The softball team was tied for first place in the YMCA Sixth Grade School League, and they were scheduled to play Crockett that day immediately after school at the softball diamond of Sam Houston. Most of the players were in this class. Now they would have to forfeit the game and would not get to play for the city championship the following week. Ronnie felt terrible, and then he began to blame the three who had misbehaved. Two of them were starters on the softball team.

About thirty minutes later, Ms. Berry came on the loudspeaker and said that the softball players in Ms. Birk's sixth grade class could come to her office after school, get a whipping, and then play in the softball game. Ronnie was elated. Then he got to thinking about getting his first whipping at school, and it was not all positive, but they would still get to play the game, which was more important.

Minutes before school let out, Ms. Berry came on the loudspeaker a third time and said that all students in Ms. Birk's sixth grade class who had all As in conduct for the year would not have to stay after school. She announced the names of those who had all As in conduct for the school year. Noel Crenshaw and Ronnie were the only boys that she named. Noel did not play on the softball team. To this day, Ronnie thinks that Ms. Berry looked for a legitimate way to give him a way out of getting punished, and like Shelby, he always tried to be a good reflection of Mother in his conduct. Mother was always a good example of proper behavior.

When school was out, Ronnie got his ball glove and went directly to the softball diamond. He was the first player to get there, and Ms. Smith came out and started talking to him. Since he was the pitcher, he was standing near the pitching rubber. She handed him the new game ball, and he started tossing it up and catching it. Neither the opponents nor the umpires had come yet. Shortly, one by one he saw his teammates coming out to the ball field. He began to think about being the only player in the class who had to stay after school who did not get a whipping and how they were going to razz him about it.

Jimmy Pitts, his best buddy except for Rod, walked by him to his shortstop position and did not say a word to him. Tony Deatherage walked by him to his position at first base and said nothing to him. One by one he got the silent treatment. Ronnie never found out what they said to the three culprits. But when the game started, they all supported his pitching with good fielding, and they were able to score more runs than Crockett. The results of the city championship game that followed were noted on page 51 in a tribute to Ms. Smith.

It was about this time that Rod and Ronnie began lifetime friendships with Bill McFall who played on the Crockett softball team. A few years later, Bill and Shelby became friends. During this softball season, Mother would pick Shelby up after school at Austin grade school and come to the games. They missed the first inning of a few games.

Because of Mother's casual acceptance of Shelby's differences from other children, he did not worry about his handicaps. He strived to do the best he could with what he had. Sometimes when children who were strangers to him would stare at him or whisper about him, it bothered Shelby some. One time he told Mother that if he could, he would have stuck his tongue out at them. But most of the time, adults and children were impressed by what they saw him doing physically, despite his handicaps. *Examples of these are included in the testimonials chapter.*

A young, small, mixed-breed dog that was so ugly in shape and color that no one would want it came to Shelby's house. Shelby got Mother to feed it daily, and it stayed and became his dog. He named the dog Chippy. Everywhere Shelby went, Chippy went with him. And Shelby frequently went somewhere.

One day Shelby and Ronnie put on the boxing gloves and started slugging away. Shelby chose to be Joe Louis, the current world heavyweight boxing champion. Ronnie was Jersey Joe Walcott. Shelby hit Ronnie on his left eyebrow with the pointed stub and lacerated Ronnie's brow. Instead of punching Ronnie with the padded glove, he hit him with the laced side. With Ronnie's brow bleeding, Shelby (alias Joe Louis) won by a TKO, but he should have been disqualified. Ronnie (alias Jersey Joe Walcott) was cheated just as Walcott was cheated in the real championship match in December 1947 against Louis. The Shelby versus Ronnie boxing matches were discontinued. That was the first of Shelby's history of hitting someone with his pointed stub.

At the end of school year 1948–49, *Shelby completed fifth grade requirements. He had made five grades in his first three years in school. Each year thereafter, he completed the requirements for one grade.*

Early May 1949, Ronnie started a special backyard baseball league named the Little Ox Baseball League. *It was especially designed to enable Shelby to play several games each week with the boys in their neighborhood.* One exception was Tommy Plemons who walked or rode his bike almost three miles to play. The games were played in their backyard with short bases, short pitching distance, short distances to outfield fences, a tennis ball, and a Louisville Slugger baseball bat that was split right down the middle. An older friend, Billy Bob Brashear, batboy for the Spudders, kept Ronnie supplied with broken bats, which could be easily split down the middle.

They usually had five players on each team, which consisted of a pitcher, first baseman, shortstop, and two outfielders. The shortstop moved closer to second base when the batter was hitting left-handed. No catcher was required. A player of the team at bat would retrieve pitched balls not hit. All right-handed hitters had to bat left-handed and vice versa.

Occasionally, a batter hit a homerun past the alley and over Mr. Box's back fence into his vegetable garden. He never complained. Either Rod or Ronnie would carefully retrieve the ball. Mr. Box was a medical doctor, and each summer he would give Jim B., Rod, and Ronnie free physical exams required for going to Boy Scout summer camp.

All the Little Ox Baseball League players except Shelby played on Kid Baseball teams, so the quality of hitting and fielding was good. Shelby played often and hit well, but he could not cover as much ground or field the ball or throw the ball as well as the others. The most important thing about this league was that Shelby got to play almost real "baseball," enjoyed it very much, and the other players felt good about that.

The reader is asked to recall the following paragraph from page 22: "Note how much of this and the prior page coverage is about Roddy and Ronnie and how little is about Shelby. That is a legitimate measuring stick of the physical activities of a normal child ages three to eight compare to those of Shelby at the same ages. And that differential remained similar for five more years."

In Ronnie's opinion, that physical activities differential was slightly less from ages nine to twenty-one, but regarding the social activities, the differential was greater, especially from ages sixteen to twenty-one. Additionally, the employment activities differential was infinitely greater for the remainder of Shelby's life. *Other than that, Shelby was competing on a level field.*

Rod began working at his daddy's service station, and Ronnie continued working at his daddy's grocery store. Rod pumped gas, cleaned windshields, and put air in tires. Their summer hours were longer, but they were always able to play their YMCA baseball games. A few mornings Daddy let Ronnie open the store before he got there.

One such morning, a lady came in and said her husband wanted some pork chops for breakfast. She asked for four pork chops. Ronnie said okay and did not tell her that he had never cut pork chops from a pork loin. However, he put Daddy's butcher apron on (way too big), put the pork loin on the butcher block, cut down to the bone with the very sharp butcher knife, sawed through the bone with the butcher saw, put the chops on butcher paper, put a box below the raised butcher scale, got on the box, stood on his tiptoes, weighed the chops, wrapped them in butcher paper, taped it, put them in a sack, took her money, and thanked her for coming in. No one ever complained about his butchering.

Even though he worked in his dad's grocery stores until he was eighteen, that is the only time he used a butcher knife except to cut slices off a big round of longhorn cheese. Shelby never used a butcher knife, much less a butcher saw, but Ronnie would bet he could find a way to do it.

At age twelve, Rod and Ronnie became Boy Scouts. In mid-June, they went with Jim B. to Boy Scout Camp Perkins near the Red River for one week, but Shelby stayed home. It was the second camp for their best friend Jim B., and he *showed them the ropes*. They slept in tents, swam in a cool pool that was downstream from a spring-fed lagoon for boating and canoeing, hiked, worked on merit badge requirements, pitched horseshoes, and enjoyed every minute of it. Ronnie sent two postcards[1] to Shelby.

At age thirteen, Shelby became an active Boy Scout. Their scoutmaster, Mr. Nate Gould, came to their house weekly and worked with Shelby on his scouting requirements. Ronnie remembers them working on learning and using Morse code. The first merit badge he earned was "music." But Shelby was not capable of going to summer camp. His special needs could not be met even with the help of Rod,

Jim B., and Ronnie. Also, his participation in many of the activities would have been limited.

Rod and Ronnie played on the Greyhounds in the YMCA Kid Baseball Midget League and were undefeated city champions. A few of their games were competitive, but they also won by scores of 35 to 1, 30 to 2, and 19 to 2. All their players were students at Sam Houston. Shelby was the Greyhound batboy and enjoyed every game. As each Greyhound batter hit the ball and ran to first, Shelby ran to grab the bat and take it quickly to the dugout. The baseball expression for that is "jerking the bat." He jerked a lot of bats that season, and he was a hit with the opponents and the fans. In early August, the four league championship games were played in Spudder Park, the home of the Wichita Falls Spudders professional baseball team. In the Midget League game, the Greyhounds were losing by a score of 3 to 7, mainly because of three errors, but they came back strong to win 13 to 7. A large crowd got to see batboy Shelby in action, and as usual, he got along well with the plate umpire.

The mothers of the Greyhounds players had dyed denim jeans black for each of the players and sewed a white stripe down the outside of each pant leg. That matched their black T-shirts with white lettering of "Greyhounds" and the white greyhound image and black baseball caps with a white "G." They also wore black and white baseball stockings below their knee-length pants. The homemade uniforms were commended in the *Wichita Record News*'s article about the game the following morning.[2]

Shelby and Ronnie followed the Spudders closely starting in July 1949 because they were leading the Big State League, and they had a catcher, Frank Saucier, who was hitting better than any player in professional baseball. When the regular season ended, the Spudders had the best record, but they lost to the Waco Pirates in the playoffs, four games to two. Saucier won the Louisville Silver Slugger Award for Minor Leaguers with a batting average of .446. Peterson, Shelby's favorite pitcher, won twenty games, and McCarty, his favorite hitter, led the team in home runs.

In the 1949 World Series, the Brooklyn Dodgers with strong fan support from Shelby, Rod, and Jim B. could only win one of their five games against Ronnie's New York Yankees. In Texas high school football's highest classification, the WFSH Coyotes won the state championship. Shelby was as proud of the Coyotes as Rod and Ronnie were.

Starting with school year 1949–50, Mrs. Willams took her class on a field trip each year. Ronnie remembers three of them because he was invited to join them when Mother took some of the students in her car. The first year the class went to Spudder Park to see the Ringling Bros. and Barnum & Bailey Circus set up the huge tent using the labor of elephants as well as men. Then they walked down the line of caged trailers while looking at all the animals including lions, tigers, monkeys, and others. Finally, they watched the clowns, trapeze artists, lion tamers, elephants, and others perform in the three-ring shows.

The sixth grade began to be more of a challenge to Shelby than the first five grades. He could no longer draw on knowledge that he had acquired by following the schoolwork of Rod and Ronnie the year before. Last year while they were doing sixth grade work, he was busy doing fifth grade work and did not have time to learn what they were learning. But Ronnie does not remember him asking for help with his homework.

One of Shelby's subjects was Texas history. He had already read through the Magnolia Mobil Oil Company's *Texas History Movies Book* that Ronnie was given a year earlier. That gave him a head start. He probably received his own copy in the sixth grade. In any event he made an A in Texas history.

Mrs. Williams taught Shelby how to read sheet music while he was playing the melody on the school piano with his right stub. His left stub was too large to play a single piano note. She also gave him assignments to read music while playing his piano at home. Later she encouraged Mother to get a marimba for Shelby to learn to play. She thought it would be the best musical instrument for him to learn to play well with his stubs. Her suggestion led to Shelby's favorite activity for the rest of his life.

She also said that the boot maker that made Shelby's special shoes could make him leather cuffs to fit his stubs and hold his mallets. Mother was able to purchase a new marimba at McCarty Music Store for $400.[3] It was a model 8-366-X Rosewood Vintage 3-octave marimba manufactured by Ludwig. Ronnie has no idea how much the boot maker charged for the mallet holders, but they were ingenuous and well worth the price.

Shelby took to that marimba like a duck to water. He practiced at home every day, and it was amazing how fast he improved from month to month. Playing his marimba became his most enjoyable activity, and for the rest of his life, he played to bring glory to God.

Because the two junior high schools in Wichita Falls were at full capacity that school year, the seventh graders from the four grade schools with the most seventh graders stayed in their grade schools one more year. Those included Alamo, Crockett, Austin, and Sam Houston. Rod and Ronnie were happy to keep the same teachers for another year.

They continued with their violin lessons with Mr. Locascio and with Mike Neel played and sang "Whispering Hope" for a Parent Teachers Association meeting and for a small country church. They were musicians on stage four years before Shelby, but they performed to much smaller audiences and with less musician proficiency. Shelby practiced much more than they practiced.

Christmas 1949, Shelby got records, sheet music, music books, books, and clothes. Ronnie got a football table game, X-Acto woodcarving set, books, and clothes. The football game had a metal football field with small players mounted on metal bases that moved forward when the electric switch was turned on. Shelby could play it as well as anybody. It was best to have two or three on a team because it took time between plays to reposition the twenty-two players. David got toys and clothes.

In late February 1950, Shelby, Rod, and Ronnie went to a funeral with the rest of their families except Lee Roy and Sonny. Their friend, Douglas Box, died tragically while swimming at the YMCA pool after school with his brother Jerry, Jim B., and Rod. Douglas had dived into the pool at the deep end, swam underwater to the shallow end, touched the side near the end, got out of the pool, said, "I thought it was the end," and died instantly. He was the same age as Shelby.

Douglas, like his brother Jerry and sister Nancy, was a good person and student. He could run faster and jump higher than any of the boys in their neighborhood. He ran and jumped over the hood of a parked car when hoods were taller than now. It was the first death of a friend near their age. The Boxes moved to Dallas shortly before school year 1949–50 ended.

Rod began working after school at the YMCA, and soon Ronnie joined him in checking the boys clothes in the locker room when they came to play in the gym, swim in the pool, or use the workout room. They later checked them out when they were ready to leave. One day they were in the snack bar when YMCA director Don Greer came in with his secretary. Don introduced them to her, and she asked, "Who was born first?"

Rod answered, "I was."

She turned to Ronnie and asked, "How much later were you born?"

He answered, "Three weeks and two days." She gasped with her hand to her mouth, and Don started laughing. Rod and Ronnie did not know why he was laughing until he explained to her that they were double cousins, not twins. Then all four began laughing.

Ronnie was the pitcher, and Rod was the left fielder on the Sam Houston team that won the YMCA Tri Hi-Y Softball League Championship by beating the Alamo grade school team.

Shelby continued to make high grades in school and at the end of May was promoted to the seventh grade, which was junior high level, but he remained at Austin grade school. Rod and Ronnie also made high grades in the seventh grade and promoted to the eighth grade at Zundelowitz junior high school (Zundy).

Summer of 1950 was good and bad for Shelby and Ronnie. The Greyhound city champs team kept the same roster and moved up to the YMCA Kid Baseball's AAA League for ages thirteen to fifteen. All their players were thirteen except two who were twelve. Their opponents were made up mostly of players ages fourteen and fifteen. They lost every game that season. Batboy Shelby did not jerk nearly as many bats as the year before because they played fewer games and got fewer batters to the plate in each game than they did in 1949.

But Shelby and Ronnie had another fun-filled summer playing in the Little Ox League, which started in April. Shelby hit better, ran better, fielded better, and threw better. Everybody enjoyed it even more than the first year. There were no changes to the equipment, rules, or dimensions. Ronnie does not remember the family who moved into the Box house, but there were no problems in retrieving homers that landed over their back fence.

Uncle John, Aunt Velma, and cousin Earlene visited the Stepps in Wichita Falls for several days. Shelby got to ride around and visit with Uncle John in his truck. When they went back to Hugo, Rod and Ronnie rode in the back of the flatbed truck with no side rails. That was 210 miles of adventure. They shot Uncle John's .22 rifle and ate fresh cantaloupes, watermelons, peaches, and tomatoes. Their cousin Ivan took them to the annual Hugo Rodeo featuring the local hero Todd Whatley.[4] They stayed five or six days and then rode a bus back home. Shelby would have enjoyed it as much or more than they, but he could not be away from Mother's care.

Ronnie worked enough at Daddy's store to make five dollars each week. He saved some money and went to Huffhines Sporting Goods and bought a Winchester pump .22 rifle model 62A for $49.60. He made a down payment of $13.60 and signed a document stating that he would make eight weekly payments of $4.50. He proudly took the rifle home. For eight weeks, he tithed fifty cents at church, which left him with no spending money. But he got free food, soda pop, ice cream, potato chips, etc. at Daddy's store. Therefore, financially, he did not suffer much. One of those weeks, Daddy found out that Ronnie had a date with a girl that Daddy liked, so he gave Ronnie a five-dollar bill. When you give the tithe to God, things like that happen!

Whatever, it was worth it because Hope Hatcher and Ronnie went to the country to shoot their rifles often. Also, they went near Dead Man's Bridge on the Wichita River with Donald New many times to shoot. Ronnie still enjoys shooting that rifle in his eighties. But he never found a practical way for Shelby to shoot the rifle that would have been fun for him. So many ideas about how to help Shelby never panned out, but that was how God planned it so that his story would be more remarkable. Shelby never complained about what Ronnie was doing that he could not do.

Rod, Jim B., and Ronnie had another fun Boy Scout camp, but Shelby stayed home. However, Mr. Gould found ways to legitimately enable Shelby to complete camping and cooking merit badge requirements. But Shelby could not earn some merit badges like lifesaving, swimming, and canoeing. He spent most of his time practicing on his marimba, playing his records, and playing with Butch, Jim S., Joe, and David. He continued to be happy with his life. Except for playing his marimba, the thing he enjoyed most was kidding around and playing with his friends.

Shelby began to buy sheet music and played many of his favorite country and western songs on his marimba. From 1943 to 1950, Shelby and Ronnie listened to *The Lone Ranger*, *The Inner Sanctum Mysteries*, *Gangbusters*, and *The Shadow* each week on the radio. They called the *Inner Sanctum* program "The Creaking Door," and they liked it because "it scared them to death." Brace Beemer was their favorite voice for *The Lone Ranger*, and when they acted out the show, Shelby always wanted to be Tonto, which let Ronnie to be the Lone Ranger. Both were pleased with their role. Shelby was usually for the *underdog*. Jackie Robinson broke the color barrier in Major League Baseball playing for the Brooklyn Dodgers. He was one of Shelby's favorite players on his favorite team. Larry Doby, who was colored, broke the color barrier in the American League playing for the Cleveland Indians. He was Shelby's favorite hitter on his favorite AL team.

School year 1950–51 was a most significant year for Shelby.

Rod and Ronnie adjusted to the new environment at Zundy in the eighth grade. For the first time in school, they had a locker in a hallway to store their books, coats, etc. A combination lock was required for the locker. For many years after graduating from high school, Ronnie had dreams about not being able to find his locker or not being able to open the lock between classes, causing him to be tardy to his next class. He was never late to class, but he obviously was afraid that he might be late.

A big negative for Rod and Ronnie at Zundy was that there was no softball diamond. In their first seven grades, they played softball during recess most of the school year. Occasionally, they played softball before school, and often they played softball after school. But at Zundy, they got to play volleyball and touch football, and they made many new friends from grade schools other than Sam Houston. Shelby never mentioned outdoor recess times in his school, and he had only about twenty different students in his class during his ten years at Austin.

In Texas high school football's highest classification, the WFSH Coyotes won the state championship for the second year in a row. Again, Shelby was as proud of them as Rod and Ronnie were. Zundy beat Reagan junior high school in football, which pleased Rod and Ronnie.

Rod and Ronnie started playing football in the Boys Club Midget Football League. The age limit was 15 and the weight limit was 110 pounds. Their coach was George Washburn, former lineman for the 1949 Coyotes state champions. They chose "Eagles" for their name. On offense, Rod played running back, and Ronnie played center. On defense, Rod played safety, and Ronnie played linebacker. They practiced on a plowed field, which is now where Lawrence Road crosses Kell Boulevard. They lost more games than they won, but they had a good time wearing football uniforms, and they took a bus trip to Goree, Texas, to play a night game. Shelby and Mother came to their games that were played at Bridwell Park at night.

Rod and Ronnie still often worked for their dads after school and Saturdays. At that time, Shelby could run and jump; hit, throw, and catch a baseball; pass, catch, and kick a football; make short shots using a regulation ten-foot basketball goal; and play simulated games in baseball and football. He became the most popular baseball or softball batboy in Wichita Falls during the 1950s, 1960s, and early 1970s.

Christmas 1950 Shelby got books including *Black Beauty*, music books, records, and clothes. Ronnie got a Rawlings PlayMaker7 baseball glove, books, clothes, and a tooling leather kit for stamping belts, wallets, and bracelets. Shelby and Ronnie were always avid readers. David got a firetruck, books, airplane, cap pistol, and clothes. Rod, Butch, and Jim came to their house, woke them up, showed them some of their gifts, and watched them open all their gifts.

Mrs. Williams told a local radio station about Shelby, and they soon had him on the air. He played a few songs on his marimba and his short biography was read. That prompted Gerry Wright of radio station KWFT in Wichita Falls to interview Mrs. Williams, Shelby, and Mother and submit an article about Shelby with photos to *People Today* magazine.

Ms. Wright's article was published in the April 25, 1951, edition of *People Today* in the People of Courage section. One photo shows a sample of his handwriting, a second photo shows him writing at his desk, a third photo shows him playing his marimba, a fourth photo shows him tap dancing, and a fifth photo shows Shelby ready to hit the next pitch. Ronnie and his bat are in that photo. Joe Dimaggio, the New York Yankee hall of famer, was on the back cover of that issue swinging for the fences. The Yankee Clipper did not know what good company he was in. Shelby was pleased to be a celebrity just doing what he enjoyed best, but he would have preferred his Dodgers' Duke Snider in place of Dimaggio.

In the spring 1951, Mrs. Williams took her class on a field trip to Tom Medder's cattle ranch south of Wichita Falls. Mother drove Shelby and some of his classmates and Ronnie got to go also. They watched the cowboys on horseback cut out the young calves, rope them, tie them, brand them, dehorn some of them, and castrate some of them. Not a fun day for the calves. Most of the class felt sorry for the calves. Shelby enjoyed watching the horses, but he liked the circus field trip better.

For the first time in his life, Shelby sat on a pony and had his picture taken. A traveling photographer with a black and white pony came to their house, and Mother paid him to put Shelby in the saddle and take his picture. She had dressed him in his western attire. The photographer had chaps that he put on Shelby. He looked much more like a cowboy than Rod and Ronnie in their bib overalls on a horse in 1941. From this time forward, Shelby took advantage of any opportunity to ride a horse.

For several years, Rod and Ronnie had been hiking or riding their bicycles to the Hills, which was about two miles from their homes. It was a place on the Wichita River that had cliffs, natural drainage ditches, caves, large sandstone rocks, and rattlesnakes. One of the large rocks had the face of Frankenstein carved out in it. A winding road with some challenging slopes for bicycle riding made for some competitive events. Three or four of their friends usually went with them.

Starting in 1951, Daddy often took some of them to the Hills to play "cowboys and outlaws" on Sunday afternoons. He enjoyed running up and down the hills and ditches as much as they did. Rod, Ronnie, Butch, Jim S., Joe, David, and several others usually went. The first time Daddy took them, he got them to stand on the cliff and throw rocks at objects floating down the river. They began doing that every time they went. Daddy could throw as accurately as the best of them. Shelby could not join them in any of their activities at the Hills.

One day Shelby walked out his front door and saw Joe Hallford on top of David on the front yard lawn. Shelby hollered at Joe and started running toward him. When Joe quickly got up and ran about eighty yards to the Hallford's front porch, Shelby chased him. But because Shelby had to crawl up five steps to get on the porch, Joe was able to make it to safety inside his home. Shelby did not get to use his now famous right stub this time.

School year 1950–51 ended with Shelby promoting to the eighth grade at Austin and Rod and Ronnie promoting to the ninth grade at Zundy. They had high grades again.

Early summer 1951, local sportswriter Bob Cole held a tryout at Crockett grade school for a YMCA Kid Baseball AAA League team. Lloyd and Floyd Stone helped him by notifying selected players from all parts of Wichita Falls about the tryouts. Four former Greyhounds, Jimmy Pitts, Howard Franklin, Johnny Crunk, and Ronnie made the team and became starters at shortstop, first base, left field, and second base.

The team name was Broncos, and they finished the season as undefeated champions. They won the championship game at Spudder Park 18–4. Shelby was not the batboy that first year with this new team, but he and Mother came to most of the games. It was Ronnie's first time to play organized baseball without Rod, who did not play baseball that summer. Rod worked all summer with his daddy, but they did go to Boy Scout camp together again.

Looking back now, Ronnie thinks that teams should have been formed by players from the same school district as were the Greyhounds team of 1949. The Broncos team had an unfair advantage over the other teams in 1951 and 1952. No one came close to beating them. They won one game by 35 to 1. That was not good for either team or the fans. In sports, a team or individual improves faster by playing stronger competition. However, the Greyhounds of 1949 had won by scores of 35 to 1, 30 to 2, and 19 to 2 while all players were from Sam Houston. That spoke well of the baseball prowess of that part of town.

Uncle John and Aunt Velma came for a three-day visit. Shelby enjoyed visiting with them and watching Uncle John beat Daddy in checkers. Of course, Uncle John took Shelby for several rides in his truck. Ronnie went back to Hugo with them and enjoyed their country living for six days. Aunt Velma cooked good meals with plenty to eat. Ronnie helped her pick fruit and vegetables, slop the hogs, and draw the water from the well.

Aunt Velma always made a good effort to make Ronnie's visits enjoyable, but it was a challenge this time because he had no one to play with. Norita Cody's family had moved to Fort Worth. John and Velma took him to a Henry Fonda movie in Hugo one night. The title was *The Return of Frank James*, and the story was about Frank James getting revenge by killing the Ford brothers who had killed Frank's brother Jesse. Most days Ronnie roamed Rose Hill hunting squirrels. One day he shot two water moccasins with one bullet. They were lying in a small clear stream on Mr. Cody's property, and one was lying across the other. He shot where their bodies intersected. The day before he went home, Aunt Velma and cousin Earlene took him to a public swimming pool in Paris, Texas. He had a lot of fun there. The next day, he returned home by bus while reading the latest edition of *The Sporting News*. Shelby missed a lot of these kinds of experiences.

Shelby and Ronnie continued to read the sports section of the newspaper and followed the Spudders, Indians, Dodgers, and Yankees. They listened to some of their games on the radio. The favorite Cleveland Indians players for both Shelby and Rod were Bob Feller, Bob Lemon, Al Rosen, and Larry Doby. Their favorite Brooklyn Dodgers were Don Newcombe, Duke Snyder, Gil Hodges, Jackie Robinson, and Pee Wee Reese. Ronnie's favorite Yankees were Joe Dimaggio, Yogi Berra, Phil Rizzuto, Vic Raschi, and Allie Reynolds.

Shortly after his fourteenth birthday, Ronnie passed the written and driving tests and got his driver's license. At that time, Daddy had a 1940 Chevrolet coupe, which was easy to park and drive. Ronnie was eligible at fourteen because he made deliveries for Daddy's grocery store. But he had to sit on a thick cushion to drive. Rod did the same because he picked up and returned vehicles serviced at his daddy's service station. Shelby was never able to get his driver's license, but more than once, he drove Daddy's car with help from David (more about that later).

* * * * *

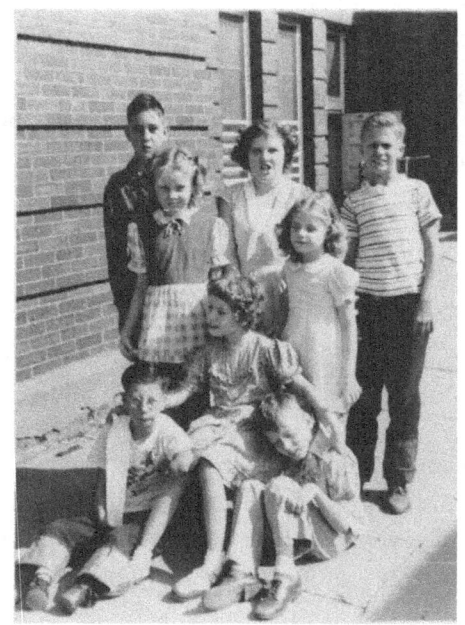

Shelby's Class in 1949

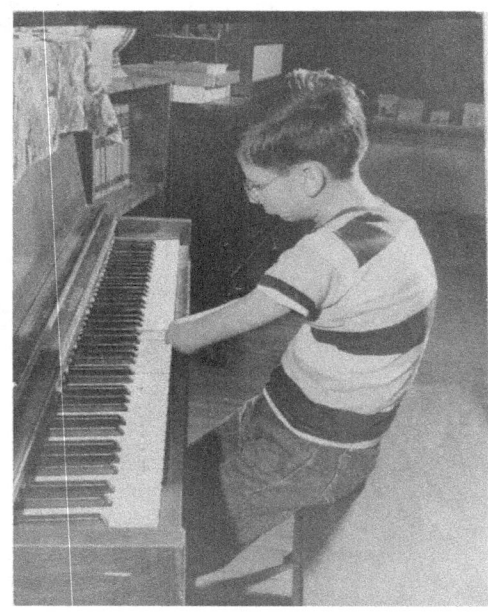

Shelby at piano in 1950

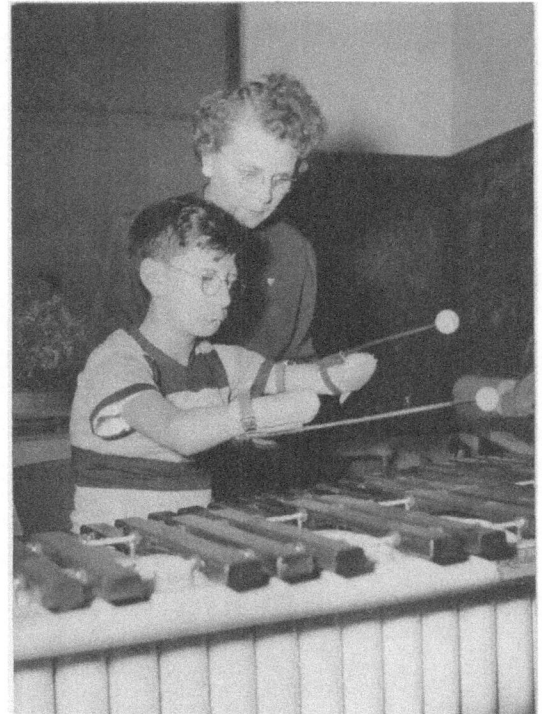

Shelby and Mrs. Williams at Austin Grade School in 1950

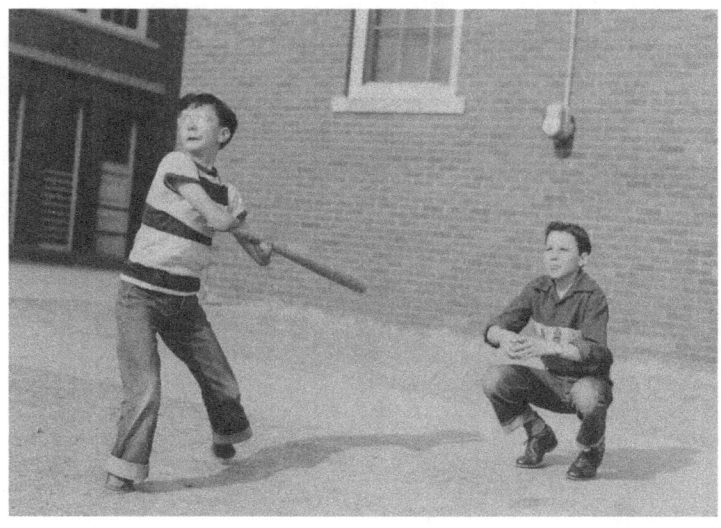

Shelby and Ronnie at Austin Grade School in late 1950

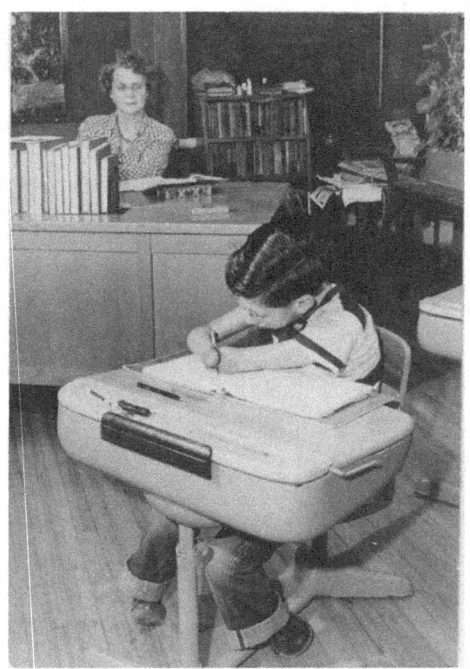

Shelby and Mrs. Williams in late 1950

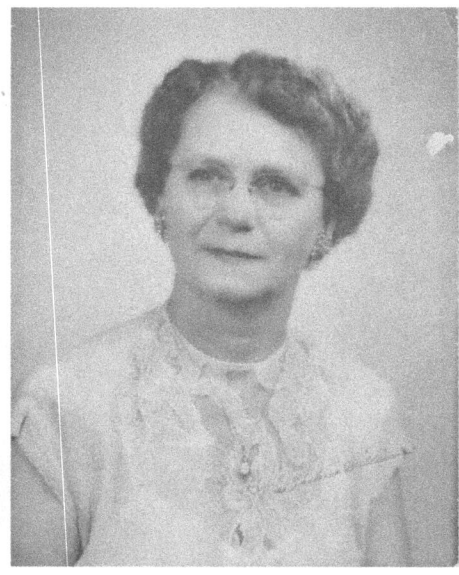

Mrs. Williams circa 1950

AN INCREDIBLE BOY AND A REMARKABLE MAN

1. Message on one of the postcards: "Dear Shelby, I wish you could be out here. I was the first one to go to sleep last night. Rod, Jim and I went up in the hills this morning and played 'Ditch 'em.' It is now 7:30am. In thirty minutes, we will go to breakfast. See you later. Ronald"
2. From the *Wichita Daily Times*, page 12, Wednesday, August 24, 1949:

    > One of the cleverest bits of ingenuity we've run across in a long time was brought to our attention during the recent Kid Baseball playoffs when we remarked that we thought the Greyhounds team was the best dressed (they had pants and jerseys to match) we had seen.
    >
    > The explanation was that mothers of the various team members had dyed the regular blue denim pants black and then sewed a strip of white material down the sides. This made the jeans match the regular T-shirts the youngster wore, which were black with white stripes down the sleeves and white lettering. Each youngster wore white-and-black sox to match the rest of the uniform.

3. Mother began ironing clothes for additional income. This enabled her to make the monthly payments for the marimba. She later had so many clients that she had to purchase a commercial ironing press, and she continued this work until 1990. She used much of her earnings providing "extras" for her sons.
4. In 1947, Todd Whatley won the steer wrestling world title and by virtue of winning more money than any other contestant in two or more events was awarded the first All-Around Cowboy title by the Rodeo Cowboys Association.

CHAPTER 4

Late Teen Years: Fifteen to Twenty (1951–56)

Shelby was at junior high school level in the eighth grade in school year 1951–52. Mrs. Williams had lost her husband. It still amazes Ronnie that Mrs. Williams could teach all required subjects from first grade to twelfth grade. In addition to math, English, music, and history, Shelby was now taking Spanish. Although his schoolwork was getting more challenging, he continued to make high grades. Shelby continued improving his skills playing his marimba at home and occasionally playing in the worship services at HHBC. He also began to sing in the church choir.

Rod and Ronnie were in the ninth grade at Zundy taking algebra, general science, English, history, mechanical drawing, and violin. They continued to make high grades, were active in their church, and continued reading many books. They had a new violin teacher, Mrs. Haseltine, who played the violin in the Wichita Falls Symphony Orchestra and served as assistant concertmistress. Unfortunately, they lost contact with Mr. Mike Locascio who had gone back to active duty as a captain in the US Air Force.

The Dodgers played a best of three game series with the New York Giants for the National League pennant. The Dodgers had blown a thirteen-game lead in August. Then in the third game of the playoff series, Bobby Thomson of the Giants hit his famous ("infamous" to Shelby, Rod, and Jim B.) walk-off homerun to win the pennant. That homer was called "The Shot Heard Around the World," but Ronnie heard it in mechanical drawing class because his teacher, Mr. Williamson, was listening to the game on his radio while the class worked on a drawing assignment. Ronnie did not feel sorry for Rod or Jim B. because they ganged up on him, but he did feel sorry for Shelby because his Dodgers could never be world champs.

The Yankees won the American League pennant. Then they beat the Giants in the World Series. Joe Dimaggio was still Ronnie's favorite player, but he was getting interested in the young Mickey Mantle. The Yankees had also won the World Series in 1947, 1949, and 1950. The Cleveland Indians won the World Series in 1948 for Shelby and Rod. Shelby sometimes seemed to like Rod more than Ronnie in some areas of life.

Shelby diligently continued to play his marimba daily and broadened his scope of music genres. His three favorite genres were Baptist church hymns, classic country, and southern gospel, but he also played western, classical, Christmas, and pop music.

Rod and Ronnie started going to the Kemp public library to check out books. They liked biographies, *Hardy Boys* mysteries[1] by Franklin W. Dixon, and books about baseball and football. Also, they bought a few books at Lovelace Bookstore downtown. Shelby read some of the books that Ronnie brought home.

Rod and Ronnie played football again in the Boys Club League. Their coaches were Jimmy Lawrence and David Cox. Jimmy was a running back on the 1949 Coyotes state champion team. Their team name was Demons. Rod played end on offense and halfback on defense while Ronnie played center on offense and linebacker on defense. Lloyd and Floyd Stone, friends of Rod, Ronnie, and Shelby, also played in the backfield. Shelby came to all their games and some practices.

During practices at Bridwell Park, an older teenager came out regularly to watch the Demons. It became obvious that he was mentally impaired. Several of the Demons went out of their way to make him feel useful. For example, they would ask him to retrieve footballs that accidentally left the field of play. He was often standing on the sidelines with one of their practice balls in his hands, ready to give to a coach or player when it was needed. He was nicknamed Hoss, and it became obvious that it pleased him.

One of the referees was a young man who because of his size looked more like a jockey than an official. He told the Demons to call him Corky. He always wore official referee attire in the games and took pride in his job. He moved quickly with jerky motions, and his speech was often difficult to understand, but Rod and Ronnie encouraged their teammates to treat him with respect.

The Demons were undefeated until they lost the championship game. Rod, Floyd, Lloyd, and Ronnie made first team on the All-Stars, and the All-Stars beat the Champs. Shelby, Mother, and Ruby came to all the Demons games, which were night games at Bridwell Park, except both the league championship game and the Champions versus All-Stars game were at Coyote Stadium in the afternoon.

Rod and Ronnie started dating girls occasionally. Most of Ronnie's dates were with Janice Hallford. Shelby did not have a girlfriend. Rod and Ronnie continued working for their dads, but Shelby did not have an opportunity to work for pay

Shelby and Mother took a trip, and Shelby sent Ronnie a postcard from Saint Louis dated October 13, 1951. What he wrote said a lot about what news from back home was most important to him: "Dear Ronnie, we had a wonderful time today sightseeing for two hours. What was the final score of the Wichita Falls Coyotes vs the Denison Yellowjackets? Bye. Love, Shelby"

Mr. John J. Lucas, who was courting Mrs. Williams, gave Shelby an autograph book on October 15, 1951. In the fly leaf, Mr. Lucas wrote,

> Presented to
> Shelby R. Stepp
> By
> John J. Lucas
> Oct. 15, 1951

AN INCREDIBLE BOY AND A REMARKABLE MAN

On the first page, he wrote,

> Today I had a wonderful joy,
> In the form of a letter from a boy.
> I have never seen his face,
> But I know his soul is full of grace.
> One whom I know I can love
> Sent to me from God above.
> John J. Lucas

Mrs. Williams wrote,

> My Dear Little Boy,
>
> To have worked and known you has been one of my life's greatest joys. Your noble Christian life has been an inspiration to me to be a better woman.
> God bless you and keep you always the same sweet, noble, lovable boy that you are.
>
> Devotionally yours,
> Mrs. Thelma G. Williams

Mother, Uncle Ike, and many others wrote in it in 1951 and later.

Christmas 1951. The early morning wake-up was made by Rod, Butch, and Jim at the home of Shelby, Ronnie, and David. Shelby got records, music books, books, and clothes. Ronnie got clothes, books, and a tabletop football game with a lighted surface. The player who was on offense selected and inserted an offense template. Then the player on defense inserted a defense template. Neither player knew what template was selected by their opponent. Then the player on offense slowly pulled a tab on the tray that contained the two templates, and the light showed each play developing and the result of the play. Shelby could easily play that game. David got toys, books, and clothes. Ronnie gave Mother two new chenille bedspreads.

In the spring 1952, Mrs. Williams took her class to the Memorial Auditorium to see Gene Autry sing on stage. Mother and Ronnie got to join them. Shelby got to hear his favorite Hollywood Western cowboy sing live. As Ronnie remembers the event, Gene Autry rode his horse Champion onto the stage. After the performance, Shelby's class got to meet and talk to Gene Autry. Ronnie stood and watched from the back of the room. Gene was good with the children.

One month later, Rod and Ronnie played their violins with the Wichita Falls Symphony Orchestra in that same Memorial Auditorium. All the students taking violin in the two junior high schools were invited to a rehearsal with the orchestra. They practiced the song "Roses from the South" by Johann Strauss II, and two nights later, they played that song with the orchestra before a large audience. Shelby, Mother, and Aunt Ruby were in the audience. Ronnie remembers when the conductor directed them to bring their violins up to the ready position, as he raised his violin to his chin, he heard the rattles[2] inside the body of his violin sweep across the floor of the body. The sound seemed louder than usual, but no one in the audience could tell where it came from if they did hear it. Everyone said later that the students played well.

Shelby attended the performances of the Wichita Falls Symphony Orchestra occasionally from 1960 to 2000. Sometimes he rode his three-wheeler, which he got for Christmas in 1962.

At the end of school year 1951–52, Shelby was promoted to the ninth grade while Rod and Ronnie were promoted to the tenth grade at Wichita Falls Senior High. All three had high grades again. The Little Ox Baseball League was still a fun time for them primarily because of Shelby being able to play. But this was its final season. They had reached the age where boys had more choices about what to do with their time, and they began playing more league games in multiple sports. One of the major choices was spending time with girls. But Mother did not encourage Shelby to pursue that choice.

While Jim S. and David were on the front porch sparring playfully, Shelby walked out, and thinking that almost nine-year-old Jim was hurting six-year-old David, he hit Jim in the eye with his right stub (the pointed one). Jim quickly turned and ran home. Then David explained to Shelby that they were just playing; Shelby felt bad and later apologized to Jim. That was the second of Shelby's history of hitting someone with his pointed stub. Jim still talks to this day about how bad that punch hurt him.

At this time, Mrs. Thelma Williams married Mr. John J. Lucas and became Mrs. Thelma Lucas. This marriage did not affect her relationship with Shelby as his teacher and as his friend, and Mr. Lucas befriended him.

Shelby and Ron continued to follow the Spudders by reading the newspaper sports pages and listening to games on the radio, but not as often as before. Lloyd, Floyd, and Ronnie played on the Broncos again, and they were undefeated champions in the YMCA Kid Baseball AAA League. Shelby was their batboy for the season. They won the championship game at Spudder Park by a score of 15 to 1. Jim Pitts had moved to Newcastle, Texas.

In early August, the Broncos went to the Tri-State Tournament (Texas, Oklahoma, and Arkansas) for ages fifteen and younger in Okmulgee, Oklahoma. Six players including Ronnie rode in Mrs. Stone's car with Floyd driving, and five players went by train. Their best hitter and first baseman, Howard Franklin, did not make the trip. They did not have an adult with them, and after the Okmulgee team was eliminated, they became the favorite team of the local fans. Since Shelby could not make the trip, their player who was on deck had to jerk the bats. Ron wished the fans could have seen what Shelby could do as a batboy.

In the championship game on a Sunday afternoon, a former third baseman for the Saint Louis Cardinals came early and asked to be their manager. Ron does not remember his name. The Broncos accepted his offer, and he went to his car and came back with a carton of new Louisville Slugger baseball bats. The Broncos beat a team from Oklahoma City by a score of 11 to 2 to win the tournament. That made them eligible to go to the national tournament in Chicago, but they could not get a sponsor to finance the trip. Shelby would not have been able to go with them if they had gone to Chicago.

School year 1952–1953. Shelby was at junior high school level in the ninth grade. He was taking some of the courses that Rod and Ronnie had taken the previous year. Ron does not remember Shelby asking for help with any of his school assignments.

Rod and Ron were in the tenth grade at Wichita Falls Senior High taking plane geometry, biology, English, typing, physical education, and violin. They had a new violin teacher, Mr. Dale Brubaker, who played the violin in the Wichita Falls Symphony Orchestra. Mrs. Haseltine had moved to Tucson, Arizona. They worked for their dads when they could. They dated some, but Shelby did not date. Church was still important in their lives. They attended all Sunday and Wednesday services, Sunday school before the morning worship service, and Baptist Training Union before the evening service.

In the 1952 World Series, the Yankees beat the Dodgers in seven games after losing three of the first five. Mickey Mantle homered for the winning run late in both game 6 and game 7. As of 2020, only twice in the history of Major League Baseball has a team won four straight World Series. The Yankees did it both times. Lou Gehrig was the star on the Yankee teams that won the World Series from 1936 to 1939. Casey Stengel managed the Yankees in winning five World Series from 1949 to 1953.

Daddy and Uncle Sonny started construction on another concrete block building on Grant Street next to Sonny's service station. Two-thirds of the building would be Daddy's new grocery store, and one-third would be Sonny's to rent to two barbers.

The Wichita Falls Coyotes probably had the best football team in the state during the season of 1952. They were undefeated when they played Corpus Christi Ray in the state championship game, and they had allowed only thirteen points during the ten district and playoff games. But one of their buses broke down on the way to Corpus Christi, which added many hours and discomfort to their trip as well as loss of sleep. Additionally, they ate at a restaurant that was not in their itinerary, and some of the players got sick.

They arrived in Corpus Christi too late to go through their normal pregame preparation, and they took the field in a high humidity environment instead of the dry air to which they were accustomed.

They wore down in the second half and lost the game. The best team wins most of the time, but not always. Shelby and Ron listened to the game in the dining room and were sad and disappointed.

Rod and Ron played football again in the Boys Club League. They were at the limit on both age and weight and played on the Demons team with the same coaches as last year. Rod continued at the same positions while Ronnie played tailback on offense and halfback on defense. They saw a lot of Hoss at their practices at Bridwell Park, and they were friendly to him and made sure he had opportunities to help the team. They had a good year with only one loss, but again, that loss was in the championship game. Rod and Ron made first team on the All-Stars again, and the All-Stars beat the Champs. Shelby came to all their games, which were night games at Bridwell Park, except one night game at Sheppard Field, and both the Championship game and the Champions versus All-Stars game were at Coyote Stadium in the afternoon.

Corky again officiated in all their games and was treated with the same respect that was given to the referees of Coyote football games. Shelby got a kick out of Corky. It was their last season of organized football except for intramural flag football at Texas A&M a few years later.

Christmas 1952, the six Stepp boys observed their early Christmas morning routine. Shelby got a bicycle with training wheels (permanently mounted while he rode it), records, music books, books, and clothes. Ronnie got a Smith-Corona portable typewriter, books, and clothes. David got a metal fort with plastic cowboys, horses, and Indians, other toys, books, and clothes. Ron gave Mother a waffle iron, but he kind of felt bad about that gift because it was partly for him. Shelby began to spend less time at home. Most of his casual time was spent at Aunt Ruby's house and yard.

At midterm at WFSH, Ron went to Mr. Richard Moss, the head coach of the Coyote baseball team, and asked to be transferred to the baseball class, which met during the sixth period of school. When asked what subject he currently had for sixth period, Ron answered that he had violin class three days and study hall two days each week. When Coach Moss asked what his parents thought about dropping the violin class, Ron said they gave him permission to transfer. Coach Moss approved the transfer, and Ron was thrilled.

A few days later, Mr. Brubaker came to Daddy's grocery store where Ron was working and told him that he would give him private violin lessons for a reasonable price. Daddy left the decision up to Ron who declined. Later Ron realized that it was one of the worst decisions of his life. He could have done baseball and violin. To this day, Ron regrets his decision. *Shelby would have done both!*

Rod worked for his dad when he could and purchased a Coke vending machine for $30 and placed it near the front door of the station. This gave him some additional income. Shelby bought Dr Peppers from Rod when he could have walked seventy feet for a free one at Daddy's new grocery store. Those Dodger fans stuck together unselfishly. Rod probably gave him most of those Dr Peppers.

Daddy and Sonny finished their building, and Ron helped Daddy move his grocery store equipment, fixtures, and inventory into his area of the building. It was just one block south of his former store. Daddy did not lose any customers and soon began to add new customers. Ron enjoyed working there even more than the other store.

In the spring of 1953, a one-week revival was held at Highland Heights Baptist Church. Ron talked Daddy into going with him one night. Mother took charge of the grocery store from 6:30 p.m. to closing at 8:30 p.m., and Daddy, Shelby, and Ron went to church. Ron was seated on the aisle next to Daddy so he could talk to him about accepting Christ as his Savior during the invitation. Shelby sang in the choir. Joe Hallford came in as the service started and insisted on sitting between Daddy and Ron. (Today Ron can see this incident playing out so vividly in is memory in color, that it is much like living it again.)

When the service moved on to the time of invitation, Ron was praying that Daddy would be convicted and go forward to be saved. For about six years, he had been deeply concerned about Daddy not being a Christian and even had several dreams where Jesus was coming back to earth, and he was running to find Daddy and pleading with him to accept Jesus as his Savior before it was too late.

AN INCREDIBLE BOY AND A REMARKABLE MAN

After two verses of invitation were sung and not being able to talk to Daddy, Ron went forward and told Pastor Robert Parr of his concern for his daddy's lost condition. Brother Parr was six feet and six inches tall and towered over Ron as he said to Ron, "He is coming!" Ron thought that he was referring to Jesus's coming again, so he began to reply, but Brother Parr said, "Ronnie, your daddy is coming forward!" Ron turned just as Daddy came beside him. Ron heard all that Brother Parr said to Daddy and all that Daddy said in response. Daddy made his profession of faith in Jesus Christ as his Savior and Lord, and Ron was elated beyond words. His thought was, *I wish Mother was here.*

Seeing it so clearly in his memory sixty-seven years later is as good as if he were viewing a motion picture of it. It is enjoyable each time he remembers it. When people came forward to express their feelings to Daddy, they also said positive things to Ron. And Shelby watched it all from the choir.

After church, Ron ran to the store and excitedly told Mother all about Daddy's salvation. She became as excited as Ron, and they praised God. Then Ron got on his bicycle and rode down to the Hallford's house to tell Chester and Faye the good news. It was the happiest moment in his life to that point. The next day at Coyote baseball practice, Ron told several of the players about his daddy's conversion.

Recently, Ron reminded Joe of that night his daddy was saved and said, "Looking back, I am grateful that you sat between Daddy and me. I might have interfered with how God had planned to reach him. Thanks, Joe."

The Coyote baseball team won district and bi-district and went to the state playoffs. Lloyd was the only sophomore who made the state playoff trip where they beat Bryan high but lost to Fort Worth Polytechnic high, who won the state championship. During the season, Ron played behind four seniors at second base, got one hit in two at bats, and made several plays in the field. He does not remember Shelby coming to any of his games.

School year 1952–1953 ended with Shelby promoting to tenth grade and Rod and Ron promoting to eleventh grade. They made high grades. They continued to be active in church and Explorer Scouts, and Rod made Eagle Scout. Shelby and Ron each were awarded medals at the Annual Court of Honor. Rod and Ron worked for their dads as much as they could, and they dated occasionally.

Summer 1953, Rod, Jim B., and Ron played in the YMCA Church Youth Softball League. Jim was the best catcher in the league, Rod played second base, and Ron played shortstop. They came close to winning the championship. Shelby was their batboy.

In a big game late in the season, they were trailing by one run in the last inning. Ron was a runner on third base with one out when the batter hit a ground ball to short. Ron broke for home to score the tying run. When Shelby jerked the bat, instead of hustling back to the on-deck circle as he normally would, he stood nearby to watch Ron trying to score. Ron slid into home plate as the catcher got the throw from the shortstop, and the plate umpire called him out on a close play.

As Ron got up to walk back to the dugout, Shelby walked near home plate and kicked a lot of dirt on it. *It was an improper act by Shelby*, but the umpire casually brushed the dirt off the plate and said nothing to Shelby. After the umpire put his mask back on, Ron saw him look at Shelby and smile. He probably had seen Shelby do his usual excellent batboy duties in many other games that season. It was the only time that Shelby misbehaved as a batboy. They lost the game by one run.

In YMCA Kid Baseball, Lloyd, Floyd, Jim P., Rod, and Ron played on the Riggers in the Major League and were undefeated champions. They won the championship game at Spudder Park by a score of 9 to 0. Floyd pitched a no-hitter. Shelby was their batboy. Their manager was Mr. T. L. Edmondson who was the father of Tommy Edmonson who was the star first baseman on the Coyote team that year.

School year 1953–1954. Shelby's subjects in the tenth grade were English, algebra, art, music, and biology. Mrs. Lucas continued to push him to achieve at a high level. His skills in playing the marimba and tap dancing continued to improve.

She also was instrumental in getting him on the new national TV show *This Is Your Life*. Shelby, Mother, and Mrs. Lucas were flown to New York City to prepare for the show the following night. However, the producer or sponsor replaced him just before airtime. The reason given for the change was that Shelby's multiple handicaps would be troubling for some viewers. Shelby handled the cancellation not as a setback but as evidence that the show was not in God's plan for him. It did not discourage him one bit.

Ron thought the main reason that Shelby was rejected was because of his speech impediment. The format of the show required a lot of dialogue between the host and the person being featured. Later in this story, Shelby's testimony will show why and for whom he performed with his marimba.

In the eleventh grade, the subjects for Rod and Ron were trigonometry, chemistry, English, history, and physical education. They worked after school most weekdays and Saturdays. The Coyote football team did not make the playoffs. Shelby enjoyed hanging out at Uncle Sonny's service station because Sonny often "kidded around" with him and some of his regular customers.

Shelby played his marimba daily and played more often at church on Sundays. He started singing in the church choir every Sunday morning. He did not have a strong voice, but he enjoyed singing in the choir for many years. He still visited Aunt Ruby most days, and Chippy went with him on those visits. David always had a cat at home, but Chippy and the cat got along okay.

Then another tragic event tested Shelby's will to live up to his favorite Bible verse, "I can do all things in Christ who strengthens me" (Philippians 4:13 KJV). While sitting with Chippy and Jim S. at the curb in front of Aunt Ruby's house, a car with a loud exhaust approached going too fast, and Chippy jumped up and out on the street and started barking at the car. The driver swerved toward Chippy and ran over him, and he died immediately. That intentional act by that driver both angered and saddened Shelby. He could not understand how a person could intentionally kill a dog. Shelby never had a dog after that tragic event. Ron was sad that Chippy was gone, but he was even sadder that Shelby saw it happen. But on the positive side, Shelby and Chippy had a close and caring relationship for five years.

Christmas 1953, five of the Stepp boys watched Shelby open his gifts. He got a wristwatch, which Ron fastened on his left arm, books, records, music books, and clothes. Ron got a wristwatch, two books, and clothes. David got his first bicycle, which was new, toys, books, and clothes. Rod, Butch, and Jim showed us their favorite gifts and then went back home.

In February 1954, the students, teachers, and staff of Wichita Falls Senior High (approximately 1,800 persons) gathered in the auditorium for an assembly program. They were always told who would be speaking or entertaining, but not this time.

Rod and Ron were seated on the first row on the far left. When the curtain opened, there was Mrs. Thelma Lucas, Shelby's teacher on stage seated at the piano in front of Rod and Ron. Shelby's marimba was in the middle of the stage. A school staff member at the microphone announced that Shelby Stepp, a sophomore, would be providing the entertainment. He called Shelby on stage and turned the program over to Mrs. Lucas. Ron had not been told anything about this surprise program. Most of those present did not know Shelby.

Mrs. Lucas said a few things, during the thirty-five-minute program, about the joy of teaching Shelby from the first to tenth grade, teaching him to play the marimba for four years, and what a good student he was. Shelby played familiar songs on his marimba with her piano accompaniment. He almost danced while he was playing, which he often did. Ron was so proud to see and hear him in this setting. And when he completed his program by tap dancing to a tune played by Mrs. Lucas, Ron joined the crowd in giving Shelby a standing ovation. All his life, Ron had been proud of him as his oldest brother who often did what seemed to be impossible, but this was extra special seeing his peers appreciating what Shelby was able to do despite his handicaps.

AN INCREDIBLE BOY AND A REMARKABLE MAN

In July 2020, Jim Booher, who sang in the high school choir and played on the Coyote baseball team, shared this about that performance:

> Ron, I remember, and it was a spectacular performance that all of us from the Sam Houston School area were proud of because we had grown up with Shelby. I remember the first time I saw him tap dance I thought he had surpassed us all because of his determination with his multiple handicaps.
>
> Jim Booher

In high school baseball, Ron started at second base all but one game for the season. They beat Abilene, their biggest rival, twice and won district. Then they played Odessa high school in a three-game series in the bi-district to determine which team would make the state playoffs. In the first game played in Odessa, the Coyotes pitched their best pitcher, Gary Greenwood, and Odessa started their best pitcher, Carl Schlemeyer.[3] The Coyotes won the first game by a score of 3 to 2. Odessa came to Wichita Falls the following Saturday and beat the Coyotes in the first game 3 to 0 in a pitchers' duel between the same two pitchers. That was the first loss of the season for the Coyotes. Twenty minutes later, the deciding game started, and Odessa won 9 to 7 in a slugfest. Since the Coyotes only had to win one game of two, they probably should have saved their best pitcher for the second game. So close, but no state tournament for them that year.

School year 1953–1954 ended, and all three made high grades and got promoted. Next school year, Shelby would be a junior and Rod and Ron would be seniors.

Summer 1954 was a banner season for them in church softball and Kid Baseball. Their Highland Heights Baptist Church youth softball team were the undefeated champions of the YMCA Church Youth Softball League with seventeen wins and no losses. They scored a lot of runs, and Shelby had a busy season as their batboy.

Lloyd and Ron were employed by the YMCA as umpires for the Kid Baseball games in the three leagues for ages below sixteen. They did not umpire a single game together until the championship games at the end of the season.

In the Major League (ages sixteen and seventeen) of the YMCA Kid Baseball program, Lloyd, Floyd, Jim Pitts, Rod, and Ron played on the Riggers team. Shelby was their batboy, and they kept him busy in each game as they scored often. They were coached by Mr. Homer Miller who had played baseball with Ron's future father-in-law Webb Curfman in the early 1940s. The Riggers were undefeated and won the championship game at Spudder Park by a score of 10 to 1. This was their last year to be eligible to play in the Kid Baseball program. Lloyd and Ron umpired the Midget League and Triple AAA League championship games. Ron was plate umpire in the first game, and Lloyd was plate umpire in the second game.

Gene Stewart, a longtime, older friend of Ron, enlisted the umpires for the YMCA sponsored baseball and softball leagues. He called Ron to ask if he and Lloyd could umpire two high school girls' softball games the next day. Ron checked with Lloyd and then called Gene and told him that they could. In the first game, Ron umpired behind the plate, and Lloyd umpired the bases. In the second game, they switched umpire positions. All the players wore short shorts, and there were some nice figures among the girls from both the Burkburnett and Wichita Falls teams. Lloyd and Ron really enjoyed both games. Unfortunately for them, these were the final two games of the season for that league. Ron should have taken Shelby to watch those girls hit, run, and slide, or he could have volunteered to be batboy for one of the teams. Shelby would have enjoyed either case.

Rod bought a black 1940 Ford sedan, and he regularly drove around five or six drive-in restaurants at night with Ron and two or three other boys. He got his gasoline cheap at his dad's service station. Ron borrowed Daddy's 1950 Chevrolet sedan often and had to pay twenty-five cents per gallon for gasoline.

In August, Daddy bought the house at 2803 York Street, which was next to Uncle Sonny's service station. Shelby and Ron were not in favor of the move, but it was more convenient for Daddy. The back of the lot of his grocery store was behind the back of the lot of their new home. It was also more convenient for Shelby to visit Uncle Sonny and Rod at the service station, which he did often.

School year 1954–1955, Shelby had classes in English, advanced algebra, music, and history. Rod took Shelby to and from school in his Ford except during high school baseball season in March, April, and May. Ron rode along with them.

Rod and Ron took an advanced mathematics course, which included learning how to use a slide rule. Each student was required to purchase a K+E Log Log Duplex Decitrig Slide Rule.[4] Early in the course, their teacher required them to make a simple slide rule out of venetian blinds, log paper, rubber bands, and glue. He did that so they would better understand the basic concept of a slide rule. Rod and Ron used their slide rules in college, but afterward, it was soon replaced by calculators and then by computers. Shelby could not use a slide rule, and any ideas of how to enable him to use it, Ron deemed to be impractical. The other subjects for Rod and Ron were English, physics, solid geometry, and physical education.

On September 25, 1954, Lee Roy and Stella had their fourth son and named him Steven Dale. He was called Stevie, and later he was called Steve.

On October 27, 1954, Brother Parr, pastor of HHBC, wrote the following in Shelby's autograph book:

> Dear Shelby,
>
> It has been a real blessing to know you and to have the joy of using your ability and talent in our worship services.
> May God's blessings be eternally upon you.
>
> Affectionately Yours,
> Robert E. Parr

The Coyotes football team had a decent season with five wins, one tie, and three losses, but that record was not up to par for their high school. Shelby went to most of the home games, and Rod and Ron went to all the home games. In basketball, the Coyotes won district and bi-district, but they lost in the regionals. All three of the oldest Stepp boys went to most of the home games.

Christmas 1954, Rod, Butch, and Jim got up early, opened their gifts, and walked two blocks to the other Stepp house. They woke them, showed them their best gifts, watched them open their gifts, visited a while, ate cookies, drank cocoa, and went back home.

Shelby got a radio, music books, records, and clothes. Ron got books, a Rawlings Playmaker Supreme Stan Musial baseball glove ($29.95, a fortune at that time), and clothes. David got toys, books, and clothes. Stevie got what most three-month-old boys get for Christmas. At this time, seven Stepp boys observed their Christmas ritual.

While researching his Shelby keepsakes in 2006, Ron found Shelby's 1955 diary, which had daily entries from January 1 to September 1. *Many of his entries are quoted below.*

> Over TV this afternoon, I watched the 66th Annual Tournament of Roses Parade from Pasadena, California. (Saturday, January 1)
>
> After school I came home and went to get a coke at the store and then went over to see Sonny and his gang at the station. (January 4)
>
> Mr. Gould (Scoutmaster) came over this evening and helped me on the Music Merit Badge. (January 5)
>
> I am listening to my radio while writing in this diary. My daddy is sitting opposite to me making notes from the Bible. (January 6)
>
> [Uncle] John Stepp came down (up from Fort Worth) this evening. He took me with him (in his truck) to see Aunt Era. We stayed about an hour and a half. He is going to spend the night with us. (January 7)

> Darrell and I went to the show at the Grant St. Drive-In. We saw two good movies. (January 8)
>
> I didn't think we would make it to church because of the snow last night. But my mother helped to get me there and back. (January 9)
>
> Ruby took me to school this morning due to the ice on the sidewalks. Rod came after me this afternoon. (January 10)
>
> Tonight I listened to the Coyote-Highland Park basketball game on the radio. The Pack opened their District play with a 80 to 46 win. Their record is 11-2. (January 11)
>
> I stayed up until midnight getting my homework. I had 83 questions to answer for a history test. Brother, was it hard! (January 12)
>
> Tonight I watched Sid Caesar put on one of the best shows that he has presented on TV as long as I have watched him. (January 13)
>
> Tonight I saw on TV Sugar Ray Robinson lose on a unanimous decision to the underdog Ralph "Tiger" Jones. (January 19)
>
> Tonight I heard one of the best Coyote basketball games in ages. The Pack edged Austin in the last seconds of the ball game 48 to 47. Floyd Stone was the top scorer for the Coyotes with 16 points. (January 21)
>
> Tonight Darrell and I went to the Grant St. Drive-In. The movies were "King Richard and the Crusaders" and "Man Without a Gun." (January 22)

Ron wished Shelby had more entries about what he did in the mornings and afternoons.

> I stayed up until 11:30 PM tonight reading the book, "Gone with the Wind." (January 24)

> I got my report card today. My grades for the first semester were two B's and two C's. (January 25)

He was beginning to get complacent about his studies.

> Mr. Gould came over after a week of absence. He looked over my written work of American music. It was alright. (January 26)
>
> I sat up for a long time tonight reading "Gone with the Wind." (January 31)
>
> Darrell invited me over to listen to the phonograph records he bought this afternoon. (Tuesday, February 1)
>
> I went over to Mrs. Lucas" house to hear her records of classical music. I spent about three hours over there. (February 2)
>
> I stayed home nearly all day reading "Gone with the Wind." I am on page 707. The book has 862 pages. (February 5)
>
> This afternoon I went downtown to the Kemp Hotel to be auditioned for the Horace Heidt Show which is coming to the Memorial Auditorium on February 17th. (Sunday, February 6)
>
> Tonight I finished "Gone with the Wind." It was a good book. (February 7)
>
> I made a book report on "Gone with the Wind."(February 8)
>
> I passed my Music Merit Badge today. I certainly was thrilled over it. (February 9)
>
> Tonight at the [Annual Boy Scout] Court of Honor [at Grant St. Methodist Church], I was happy to receive a Four-Year Star and a Music Merit Badge. I also played a marimba solo. (Sun. February 13)

> Mr. Gould came over to help me with the First Aid Merit Badge requirements. (February 16)

Ron does not remember Shelby being selected to perform in the Horace Heidt program on February 17. He would have an entry in his diary if he had.

> I went to Lawton [Oklahoma] tonight and played a marimba solo for the Rebekah Lodge. (February 22)
>
> I watched the fights tonight [on TV]. Kid Gavilan lost a unanimous decision to Hector Constance [Gavilan was one of Shelby's favorite fighters]. (February 23)
>
> I stayed home and studied for three hours. (Thursday, February 24)
>
> I saw two great movies at the Grant St. Drive-In. They were "South Sea Woman" and "Distant Drums." (February 26)
>
> I went over to visit Lydia and Louis with my mother and daddy. (February 28)

Lloyd Stone, Cliff Ingle, and Ron were elected by the players to be tri-captains for the Coyotes baseball team.

> I went over to the station to see Sonny this evening. From there I went to the store and drank a Coke. (Tuesday, March 1)
>
> I sat up late tonight reading "Caine Mutiny." The time is 11:01 PM. I better be off to bed. (March 2)
>
> I went to Scout meeting tonight. (March 3)
>
> I didn't get to have my bath taken because my mother was too tired to do it after a long day's work [at the store]. She was taking Ronnie's place

[at the store] because he went to Texas A&M yesterday to stay for a couple of days. (March 5)

Rod and Ron traveled to College Station for two days of testing for scholastic scholarships to the Agricultural & Mechanical College of Texas (TAMC). They had to wait a few weeks to get the results, but they knew that they had done well.

Ronnie arrived home after a two-day visit to Texas A&M in College Station. He came about 3:45 PM. (Sun. March 6)

I played ball for a while this afternoon and after doing so I went over to the store and drank a Coke. (March 7)

Tonight I watched "The Milton Berle Show" on TV. It certainly was a good show. (March 8)

I went to Training Union [at church on Sunday evenings at 6:00 p.m.]. They had a fair program. It was based on alcohol and liquor. (Sun. March 13)

I went to the opening night of a Training Union Study Course. It was the first of five nights. (March 14)

Tonight I went to the Study Course. It was really interesting. (March 15)

Tonight the Study Course came to a close. I got a gold badge for being present every night. (March 18)

I went over to the station to see Sonny this afternoon. We talked and kidded around with each other. (March 19)

This was a beautiful day as it snowed and sleeted. Sounds good doesn't it! (March 21)

I went with my mother to help "Son"[5] [Uncle Ike] get his car home. He had a wreck but was not hurt. The other person was cut a little. (March 22)

I didn't get to go to school today because Mrs. Lucas was ill. I hated that. (March 24)"

It certainly was cold today. I had to wait for my daddy outside after school. The wind was blowing hard and the temperature was about 30 degrees. (March 25)

I went over to Darrell's house and listened to some records. I stayed for 45 minutes and then went to the store and drank a Coke. (Sat. March 26)

I had a part on the program at Training Union. I won a box of candy for giving the best reasons for why I want to be a missionary to the sick. (March 27)

Tonight Butch and I went to see "Sign of the Pagan" and "It Happens Every Thursday." (March 29)

My teacher took our class out to Sheppard Air Force Base [SAFB]. We saw different kinds of instruments for airplanes. We went inside a C-119 Bomber [a transport plane, not a bomber]. (March 31)

We arrived at SAFB at 6:30 PM. They had us eat in the Mess Hall. After that we went to an auditorium to watch a special movie. (April 1)

This afternoon we got to go through a B-36 and a Boxcar (C-119). When I arrived home this evening I was dog tired. (April 2)

This afternoon Butch, Darrell, and I went fishing. Butch caught two bass but one of them got away. (Sunday, April 3)

Happy Birthday to me. Yes, today was my 19th year on earth. I spent most of my time hanging around my ole sidekick Darrell. (April 8)

Today on TV's "Game of the Week" I watched my favorite club, the Brooklyn Dodgers, wallop the New York Yankees 14 to 5. (Saturday, April 9)

That was one of the best birthday gifts for Shelby a day after his nineteenth birthday!

After getting home from school this afternoon, I received news that somebody had flooded Ronnie Havens" car with water hoses at Sonny's station. (April 10)

Tonight I received shocking news that Sonny may have cancer in the stomach. My mother said that Rod was crying when he called. (April 11)

Tonight I went up to the Bethania (Hospital) to see Sonny. He sure did look swell. The first report says he doesn't have cancer. (April 12)

On the radio I listened to the Dodgers-Giants game. The Bums [Dodgers] won 10 to 8. (April 14)

Tonight I'm kinda cross because our television went haywire and I was unable to see the fights. My daddy was unavailable [to repair the TV] because he is staying [at the hospital] with Sonny. (Friday, April 15)

Phew! Boy, I'm really tired. I stayed on my feet [he always referred to his hands and feet] nearly all day and brother are they killing me. (April 16)

Darrell and I went to several places taking pictures. We even went down to the Grant St. Drive-In. (April 17)

I went to the revival services which are being held this week. Rev. Dean Newberry is giving the sermons. (Monday, April 18)

I went to the station and stayed with Rod until time for school. I went over and stayed with him again this evening. (April 19)

I went to the Revival and we certainly had a packed house. (April 20)

I was kinda afraid to undress and go to bed tonight because Pam, Son's daughter, was spending the night. (April 21)

I went to the Scout-O-Rama tonight and didn't get to do anything. I sure got tired. I rode home with Ruby. (April 22)

Tonight Butch and I went to see "Bridges at Toko-Ri" and "Denver to Rio Grande." (April 23)

[Uncle] John came over and ate with us before he left for Fort Worth. I certainly hated to see him leave. (April 24)

I made 95 on geometry today. That is very unusual for me. I hate the subject. (April 25)

I'm sitting here listening to "Son" tell his adventures in the Navy [during WWII]. He told such horrifying stories. (April 26)

Shelby began his job search odyssey and exercise.

This evening I went over to the Olympic Food Store to see if they could hire me. They said that I would have to see the boss tomorrow morning at 7:00 am. (Friday, April 29)

I went over to ask Mr. Ruth, owner of the Olympic Food Store, for a job, but he said that he didn't need any help. (April 30)

This evening I watched "You Are There" on television. The story was about Lou Gehrig's greatest day. The story was presented on KFDX-TV. (May 1)

I continued searching for a job this afternoon. The places were Stephens Lumber Co. and Grant St. Drive-In. (May 2)

This afternoon Mrs. Lucas took us to see Paul Harvey, the great news commentator, at the Paulk's Tire Co. [in downtown Wichita Falls]. (May 3)

My daddy came after me after school. As we were passing by the high school, we stopped for a few minutes to watch the Coyotes (Ron was practicing with his high school baseball team.). (May 5)

The Coyote baseball team won their first fifteen games of the season and only had to beat Abilene one of the two remaining games to win District. They lost the first game 8 to 3 and the second game 7 to 3. Floyd, their pitching ace, had a rib injury that prevented him from playing in either game.

In the next to last inning of the second Abilene game, the Coyotes had a chance to rally with one out and runners on first and second. Ron came to bat against the same pitcher that he had doubled off earlier in the game. He threw Ron a good pitch, which Ron hit hard, but it went on one bounce off the infield grass to the third baseman who fielded it going to his left and threw to second for the second out of the inning, and the second baseman relayed to first to complete the inning ending double play. Ron has relived that play many times over the years. If Shelby had been their batboy, Ron thinks he would have hit a line drive over that third baseman's head. It was a very disappointing season after they fielded, hit, stole bases, and pitched so well until the final week.

Uncle Sonny was diagnosed with no cancer but with numerous ulcers in his stomach. He had 80 percent of his stomach surgically removed (gastrectomy). After about a week in the hospital, he was released and told to stay at home and rest for two weeks. But he went straight to his station and even changed a tire that day. By returning straight to work, he caused damage to his stomach, which impaired healing. He was never healthy after that surgery, but he lived and worked hard for many more years. His food intake was much less than normal, and he always looked very thin. Despite that, in his remaining twenty-six years, he helped build a large sheet metal products manufacturing company[6] with the help of Uncle Louis Watkins, Rod, Butch, Jim, and Louis's son-in-law, Steve Priester.

Ron had no idea why Shelby did not have any entries in his diary about Sonny's surgery. But maybe he does. Shelby might have refused to accept that the surgery happened. Both Shelby and Sonny were stubborn about doing what they were told they could not do.

> I went out looking for a job. The places were Grant St. Pharmacy and Hudgin's Food Store. Still no luck! (May 6)
>
> I used all the roll that was in my camera. I sent them off to have the pictures developed. (May 7)
>
> My mother and I went to a Mother and Son Banquet at Grant St. Methodist Church. It was sponsored by Boy Scout Troop 6. (May 9)
>
> I received two letters today. One from [Aunt] Velma and one from "Sonny Boy"[7] [Ivan, son of Velma]. I have just written a letter to Ivan. (May 10)
>
> At lunch period Mrs. Lucas and I played for Austin students in the school cafeteria. I sure got tired and hot [the public schools had no air conditioners]. (May 11)
>
> I received the pictures that were taken last Saturday. They sure were good. I gave Rod the negatives. (May 12)

> I took care of Steve by pushing him around in his buggy. I did that for almost two solid hours. My daddy paid me a quarter. (May 14)
>
> I went to a Senior-Junior Banquet tonight. It was held at the church. (May 17)
>
> I stayed home tonight and studied history. It was about World War I. (May 19)
>
> This afternoon I played ball with a bunch of boys. They wouldn't even let my times at bat count. I hit safely seven times in thirteen tries. (Sunday, May 22)
>
> I received shocking news that I wouldn't get to pass unless I went to summer school. I certainly was sick too. (Monday, May 23)

With four days remaining for the current school year, *Shelby was shocked to hear from Mrs. Lucas that he would be required to go to summer school if he did not complete his history workbook assignments.* He began to work on it four to seven hours each day and completed it before the end of school. He was learning that regardless of how much you have achieved in the past, the challenges of learning and doing are always before you and require diligent work.

> This afternoon when I got home, I started working on my history workbook. I worked for six hours. (May 24)
>
> I worked for seven hours this afternoon and evening at home on my history workbook. (May 25)
>
> I went over to the Olympic and got two rolls of film. The man cheated me out of my money by charging me 45 cents for each instead of 40 cents. (May 26)
>
> School's Out! Yes, school is out for the summer. My mother brought my camera to take

> group pictures. One of them was of me and Mrs. Lucas. (May 27)

No summer school for Shelby after all. Mrs. Lucas used her scare tactic once more.

> I went to Iowa Park and watched the Wichita Falls Cats [semi-pro baseball team that Rod, Ronnie, Lloyd, Floyd, and Jim P. played on] play the IP team. The Cats lost 5 to 3. (Sun. May 29)

End of school year 1954–1955, Rod, and Ron made high grades and Shelby made good grades. Rod and Ron received scholastic scholarships to TAMC (it became Texas A&M University in 1963).

> Tonight I got to see Ronnie get his high school diploma. It certainly was a great sight to see. (May 31)

Rod and Ron attended the activities for the graduating seniors including a nice dinner at the Woman's Forum and the senior prom where Ron met a girl for the first time that two years later became his fiancée. HHBC also had a junior and senior banquet honoring the graduating seniors. Shelby sat next to Ron at that event.

Summer of 1955, Rod worked full-time at his dad's service station and Ron did the same at his dad's store. Earning money became more important to them since they would be going off to college in September. Shelby daily played his marimba, visited his favorite service station, bought or bummed Cokes from Rod's soft drink vending machine, read the local newspaper, played his record player, watched TV, listened to his radio, and often visited with Darrell, watched the fights on TV, went to Ron's ballgames, went to the movies, and went to church. Butch started working at his daddy's service station.

Rod and Ron played on three ball teams that summer. They played for the Jokers in the Commercial Softball League, the Highland Heights Baptist Church in the YMCA Church Men's Softball League, and the Wichita Falls Cats in a semi-professional baseball league.

Rod and Ron dated often, but Shelby did not date anyone. Jim Booher had completed one year at Texas Technological College (later renamed Texas Tech University in 1969) where he planned to earn a degree in architecture. He worked all this summer near Colorado City, Texas. Rod and Ron missed Jim a lot. Life was changing dramatically for Shelby, Rod, Jim B., and Ron.

> I went over to see Butch's new telephone setup this evening. He brought me back home just before it started pouring down rain. (Friday, June 3)
>
> Butch and I went to see "20,000 Leagues Under the Sea." Ruby came after us. (June 6)
>
> Mr. Gould came over and reviewed me on First Aid. He said he will start coming every Tuesday. (June 7)
>
> I went to prayer meeting tonight. They elected new deacons by ballots. (June 8)
>
> I was outside all day playing baseball. I sure was tired after quitting. (June 9)
>
> Tonight I saw one of the best fights I have seen on TV. Carmen Basilio won by a TKO over Tony Demarco in a 15 round welterweight match. (Fri. June 10)
>
> I went over to see Rod today because he was sick. We watched TV. (June 11)
>
> I went over at Darrell's house and listened to records with him. (June 12)
>
> Mr. Gould took me to a Doctor's house to try and pass First Aid. I did not quite catch his name. (June 14)

AN INCREDIBLE BOY AND A REMARKABLE MAN

> I got my bicycle fixed today. Rod fixed it. It had two flat tires. (June 16)
>
> This evening Ronnie and I played a little game of baseball. We pretended the Chicago White Sox were playing the Yankees. The New Yorkers won 3 to 2. (June 17)
>
> Butch, Bud Johnson, and I went to see "Man Without a Star." The second show kept me laughing all the time. It was Abbot and Costello in "Keystone Kops." (Saturday, June 18)
>
> Ronnie, Jim, and I played ball this afternoon. Jim caught, Ronnie did the pitching, and I was the batsman. (June 19)

Shelby does not mention that he hit a foul ball over the fence and cracked the windshield of a late model Buick owned by one of the barbers who rented Sonny's one-third part of the Lee Roy and Sonny building. Daddy's grocery store was in the two-third part. Daddy was very unhappy with Shelby and Ron because he had to pay for the windshield replacement.

> Butch got his driver's license today. He took me and Darrell riding. We went out to Westmoreland Swimming Pool. (June 20)
>
> I am fixing to take a bath and go to bed early because we are leaving for Hugo [210 miles from Wichita Falls] early tomorrow morning. (Wednesday, June 21)
>
> I am writing now from my Aunt Velma's which is not far from the city of Hugo, Oklahoma. (June 22)
>
> Ruby, Mother, Jim, Butch, David, Velma, Steve, and I went downtown tonight to get a jug of water and a carton of milk. (June 23)
>
> This evening Ruby, Butch, David, Velma, Jim, and I went to an old burial place. They had

steps to help get over the wall into the cemetery. It was built in 1783.[8] (June 24)

Butch and I went riding downtown this morning. We stopped at a place called "Dairyette" and bought some malts. We need them for dinner. (Saturday, June 25)

Velma invited us to her church. We went to both the morning and evening services. The pastor had me to play the piano for the evening service. (June 26)

Hooray! We're home at last. We left Hugo about 7:00 a.m. and arrived about 11:30 AM. (Butch got worried about his cat on the way home.) (June 27)

I watched Milton Berle's last show for the summer tonight. He will return to TV on September 20th. (June 28)

I sure heard a good baseball game on the radio this afternoon. The Brooklyn Dodgers beat the Giants in 11 innings on pinch hitter George Shuba's single with one out and two on base. (June 30)

Darrell and I rode with Butch in his car tonight. We went to the Seymour Drive-In. The features were "Shotgun" and "Port to Hell." They both were good pictures. (July 1)

One Friday night, all three of Ron's teams were scheduled to play. Shelby was batboy in the first game played at Hamilton Park at 7:00 p.m. The HHBC team beat First Christian 17 to 1. Then their players that also played for the Jokers in the Commercial League, drove across town to O'Reilly Park, and won that game 18 to 0. The four players that also played for the Cats missed the baseball game, which was out of town. Five nights later, Aunt Ruby took Shelby to the next Jokers game, which they won by the same score, 18 to 0.

The Youth Revival got underway today in our church. Tom Landers is the preacher and Carroll Evans is leading the singing. They will be here until next Sunday. There will be two services held Monday through Friday and at night on Saturday. (Sunday, July 3)

I went to the Fellowship which is held right after church every night. They had some ice cream for refreshment. I had two cups of it. (July 5)

I went downtown with Butch this morning and stayed for two hours. He got a Humble uniform at Muehlbergers. I got a record called "Hernando's Hideaway" by Archie Bleyer. (July 8)

At Fellowship tonight Tom Landers asked if I would play my marimba in the service tomorrow night. I told him that I would like to, but admitted that I didn't have any songs prepared. (July 9)

Tonight was the closing of another revival. Tom Landers preached on "The Day of Judgement." (July 10) [Knowing Shelby, he would have prepared and played.]

I went over to Ruby's house to watch the MLB All-Star Game. The Nationals won in 12 innings on Musial's homer 6 to 5. (Tuesday, July 12)

I went to Prayer Meeting tonight. Bro, Parr said in his message that the city council had legalized the selling of beer in stores. (July 13)

I went to (Boy Scouts Troop 6) Court of Honor and received my First Aid Merit Badge Certificate. (July 14)

After watching the Jokers drub the opposition 18 to 0, Ruby took me over to Bridwell Park to watch a concert. They played a great variety of beautiful songs. (July 15)

I went to a show this evening with Butch and Merrill Whatley. Butch took us in his family's car. We went to the Wichita Theater and saw "The Lady and the Tramp." (Saturday, July 16)

On Ronnie's little baseball set I played one of the best games yet. I knocked five round trippers [homers]. Ronnie was leading 19 to 12 after 6 innings of play. (July 17)

Darrell and I went to see "Blackboard Jungle." It started raining before it was over. Mother came and got us. (July 18)

Mother had our TV fixed. One tube had to be replaced. I got Darrell to come over tonight and watch television. (July 21)

Tonight I watched the boxing event on TV. Sugar Ray Robinson won a split decision over Rocky Castellani. He now fights Bobo Olson. (July 22)

Butch and I went to Grant St. Drive-In to see "Davy Crockett." During intermission he stayed up where there were girls. (July 23)

I spent the afternoon playing my phonograph. I did that for almost two hours. (Sunday, July 24)

Tonight I went to a softball game with Ruby. Highland Heights Baptist defeated Fain Memorial Presbyterian 3 to 2. (July 25)

I stayed home tonight and played records. It took me one hour and fifteen minutes to play my favorites. (July 26)

Tonight I got to see a real electric chair [used for executions]. Billy Mills, who has been an ex-convict for over 25 years, was the speaker at church. (Wednesday, July 27)

I heard the most shocking news in a long time. Bro. Parr is resigning as pastor of our church. I could hardly believe it when I heard the news. (July 28)

I went over to the church this evening with Darrell. When we saw his mother, she was crying. She told us why and then showed us that Bro. Parr's bookshelves were empty. (July 29)

This was the big day at the church. Bro. Parr served as our pastor for the last time. The members held a farewell party for him. (Sunday, July 31)

I went to see Highland Heights Baptist play their first playoff game against Fain Memorial Presbyterian. We won 6 to 3. (August 1)

I went over to the station this morning and talked to Rod while he was washing a car. We talked about the Cleveland Indians and Brooklyn Dodgers as usual. (August 2)

Ronnie and I played ball this morning. He hit the ball to me. We played a ballgame. I really perspired too. Sweat was all over my shirt. (August 4)

Darrell, Butch, and I went to the show at Seymour Drive-In. We saw "The Man from Bitter Ridge" and "Cult of the Cobra." (August 6)

This morning I helped Butch sweep off the sidewalks and driveways at the station. He paid me 58 cents. Brother, that's hard work. Especially in the hot sun. (August 9)

I went to Prayer Meeting tonight. They had business discussions. Darrell went with me. (August 10)

I went out to eat with Butch. We ate at Dena's Café. After that we went to car lots and looked at displays of new and used cars. (Friday, August 12)

Ronnie, Daddy, and David arrived home after spending two days at Possum Kingdom Lake. (August 14)

I took care of the bats for Highland Heights tonight. We won the championship by beating Lamar Baptist 12 to 4. (August 15)

Rod and Ron got to play on that championship team with Ron's future father-in-law, Webb Curfman, who was their best hitter. Rennie, one of Ron's best buddies, was the top pitcher in the men's league as he was the previous year in the youth's league. It was a rewarding softball season. Ron does not think their Jokers team won the Commercial League, but they came close to winning it. In the semi-pro baseball league, the Cats lost as many games as they won.

I went to Prayer Meeting and after the service I asked Mrs. Gene Shields about when we could practice our marimba and piano special for the Sunday service. (Wednesday, August 17)

This afternoon I got to practice with Betty Shields for the first time in a year. It was wonderful. I just love to practice with her. (August 18)

Darrell, Butch, and I went to see "To Hell and Back" at the Wichita Theater. It was such a packed house, we had to wait to get seated. (August 20)

Today I started playing regularly in the worship services. Betty Shields was the accompanist. This was the first time to play together in a service, and it will be the last time too. (Sunday, August 21)

Mr. Gould brought my First Aid Badge to me tonight. (Tuesday, August 23)

This afternoon a boy named Ronnie Johnson came for me to help him pass the Morse code requirements for First Class rank in Boy Scouts. (August 25)

This evening I went to see Butch because he was sick and had been for several days. I usually go to a show on this day. (Saturday, August 27)

This afternoon I went to practice the song that I was to play tonight. (August 28)

Rod took me over to Monroe St. so I could get sheet music, but the music store had moved. (August 29)

I have been bothered by a skin sore on my right hand. My mother doctored it. (August 30)

Darrell and I went to Prayer Meeting to hear a preacher from Gordon, Texas give a sermon. He certainly was good. (August 31)

My mother took me to get my new glasses. Before that she had an appointment with her dentist. (September 1) [This is the last entry in his 1955 diary.]

Because of their high marks in the scholarship exams at TAMC in May, Rod and Ron were invited to the annual freshman indoctrination camp held off-campus one week before freshman week began on-campus. They went to the camp and enjoyed it.

Ron's daily life with Shelby had ended. Shelby was not there for Ron anymore, and Ron was not there for Shelby.

School year 1955–1956 was Shelby's senior year and his last school year with Mrs. Lucas as his teacher. Because of his brief job search results, he felt that more education would be helpful after he got his high school diploma. Should he go to Midwestern University or Draughon's Business College in Wichita Falls or do a more intensive job search?

But first, he must continue to do his best in his last high school classes of English literature, economics, civics, and music. With Rod gone to college, Mother drove Shelby to and from school on most school days.

Because of Mrs. Lucas's high regard for Shelby, which she had often shared verbally to Mother and occasionally to Ron, she assisted Shelby and Mother in deciding what he should do after graduating from high school. His last year under her teaching and coaching was much like their first nine years together in that she helped him learn much more than book learning. She also guided him in planning his next few years in education and employment. However, no individual or organization ever offered good employment for Shelby.

In addition to his schoolwork, Shelby daily played his marimba, read the newspaper, listened to his radio, and did his exercises. Also, he often played his favorite records, went to the movies, watched television, visited with family and friends, rode his bicycle with training wheels, and went to church. He began playing his marimba almost weekly in church and sang in the choir.

Mother helped Daddy for several hours most days at the store, took in ironing, kept the house, and cared for Stevie who was about to be one year old. Pam Ewing, Ike's daughter, started staying at their house, and in a letter to Ron on September 12, Mother said, "Pam takes care of Steve and does a good job of it. She keeps him dry and clean." Pam was in the same fourth grade class as David, and Mother helped them at the same time with their homework. Mother also said that Ike was dating a woman who was a teacher at Wichita Falls Senior High (WFSH).

Rod and Ron were in a different environment at TAMC. They had no Reserve Officers' Training Corp (ROTC) in high school, but now they were in the Corps of Cadets under the ROTC program along with 3,400 other students, and they were living the military life 24-7. The 7,500-member student body was all-male and included many Korean War veterans. Rod and Ron made many adjustments during the first semester. The first one was wearing military uniforms every day. The second was getting their heads shaved. The third was learning to march. The fourth was memorizing campusology (facts about the buildings, traditions, statues, markers, etc. of Texas A&M).

Rod's degree plan was designed to earn a bachelor of science degree in geological engineering in four years. Ron's was to earn a bachelor of science degree in both geological engineering and petroleum engineering in five years.

They had many thrills during the Texas Aggie football season, which ended with seven wins, two losses, and one tie. This was Head Coach Paul "Bear" Bryant's second season at A&M, and he was popular with the players, student body, and former students. Rod and Ron were pleased that their Aggies beat Shelby's Baylor Bears 19–7. They would have bragging rights when they went home for Thanksgiving.

The most exciting game was at Rice. *With the Owls ahead 12 to 0 and only four minutes and fifteen seconds left in the game*, the Aggies scored from the two after a fifty-eight-yard run by Loyd Taylor and kicked the extra point to make the score 7 to 12. An onside kick by Jack Powell was recovered on the Rice 43 by Gene Stallings. On the next play, Taylor caught a pass from Jim Wright on the Owl 5 and scored untouched. The extra point was added, and the Aggies led 14–12. Shortly after Rice returned the kickoff, Jack Pardee intercepted a pass at the Owl 43 and ran it down to the 3. Don Watson ran it in for a touchdown. *Final score: A&M 20, Rice 12!*

Mother wrote that she went to see Mr. O. T. Freeman, principal of WFSH, and talked about Shelby graduating with the other seniors. Mr. Freeman assisted her in getting Shelby on the order list for his cap and gown and on the list for having his photograph taken for the 1956 *Coyote Annual*. He also assured Mother that Shelby would be seated on the stage where he could stand and walk across to get his diploma.

In a letter, Mother said that Daddy was still taking David, Jim S., Larry Slack, Joe Hallford, and David Fults to the Hills on Sundays. Daddy was fifty now, but he could run up and down those hills as good as the boys who were ten to fifteen. One-year-old Stevie got to go once.

Mother said that Shelby went to every home game to root for his Coyote football team. They easily won their first eight games but lost to Tyler 6–13 in game 9. In their final game, they beat their rival Dallas Highland Park 42–7. But Tyler also won their final game to remain undefeated and won district. Tyler won two playoff games, but they lost to Abilene 13–33 in the state championship game. Mother also mentioned that Shelby was excited about his Brooklyn Dodger team and was sure that this would be their year to win the World Series.

In Major League Baseball, the regular season ended with another New York World Series to be played. The Bronx would battle Brooklyn again. The Yankees won the first two games at home (*ho-hum*), and the Dodgers won the next three at home (*what?*). The teams went back to Yankee Stadium, and the Yankees tied the Series. (Now we got 'em!) Johnny Podres shut out the Yankees in game 7, and the Bums won the game 2 to 0 and the World Series. (Really? You gotta be kiddin' me!)

The Brooklyn Dodgers won their only World Series because Mickey Mantle had a leg injury and could hardly run. He only played in three of the seven games. During the regular season, Mantle led the American League in home runs, extra base hits, walks, on base percentage, slugging, and triples, and his speed in centerfield robbed the opponents of hits and runs. (This paragraph is for Shelby, Rod, and Jim B.)

But injuries are part of the game of baseball, and the Dodgers won the World Championship fair and square. Whoops, the "fair and square" is in question after just now reading a letter from Shelby to Rod dated October 2, 1955. In it, Shelby said, "I have been praying and asking God that if it's his will that they [Dodgers] will win a World Series, make it this year because just think this might be Jackie Robinson's and Pee Wee Reese's last year." Shelby asked for

AN INCREDIBLE BOY AND A REMARKABLE MAN

divine intervention in the outcome of a World Series. Is that fair? Considering Shelby's prayer, Ron is genuinely glad for him that the Dodgers won the World Series in 1955.

On December 1, Mother wrote that Shelby was still sick with a cold, and it was snowing and sleeting, but he insisted on going to school. When he got home, he did the same as he had for several days, he laid down and did nothing.

Shelby studied well and made good grades (one A, two Bs, one C) in the first semester of his senior year while Rod and Ron did the same at TAMC. During the Christmas and New Year's break from college, the Stepp boys were back together for almost two weeks, and they observed the early Christmas morning ritual. Ron does not remember the specific gifts, but the majority would have been clothes. Ron got a thick volume titled *The Complete Works of William Shakespeare* since he would be taking an elective English literature course in the second semester. It was good to be with family again, and Rod and Ron dated often during the holiday break.

Shelby wrote in a letter to Rod dated February 9, 1956,

> On the 25th of this month I have been asked to appear on a talent show at the U.S.O. I have not only been asked to play the marimba, but also to tap dance. Looks like another big personal appearance. Ha! Ha!

In a letter to Rod on February 26, Shelby said,

> I received your letter yesterday and was certainly glad to hear from you. Last night I had the honor and privilege of appearing on the talent show at the U.S.O. Due to the magnificent ovations in which the huge audience gave me, I had to play four more songs than I was actually supposed to play. It certainly did thrill me to receive such great responses. Furthermore, I just practically took the show away from the other performers.

On April 8, 1956, Shelby celebrated his twentieth birthday! In a letter dated April 12, Mother wrote,

> Shelby played his marimba out at the Sheppard Air Force Base tonight entertaining one of the hospital wards. He was asked and agreed to go back soon and entertain several other wards.

Shelby soon completed his senior year with good grades.

Mrs. Williams made the following entry in Shelby's autograph book:

May 25, 1956

> Shelby, Dear, so many, many things have happened in the short time that it has been my privilege to have had you in my classroom. The experience has enriched my life and inspired me more than anything has ever done.
>
> Now as you start new experiences in life, I pray God's richest blessings on you.
>
> To you always my love and prayers will be, and I will remain
>
> Your sincerest friend,
Thelma Lucas

At graduation ceremonies, he walked across the stage of the Memorial Auditorium and received his diploma with the Wichita Falls Senior High Class of 1956.

Shelby's first ten years from birth to first grade had been full of unbelievable achievements, and his second ten years from second grade to high school graduation were equally remarkable!

* * * * *

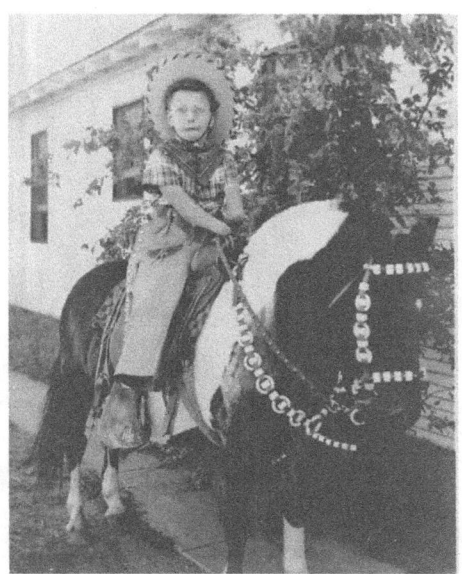

Shelby at 3105 York Street at age 15

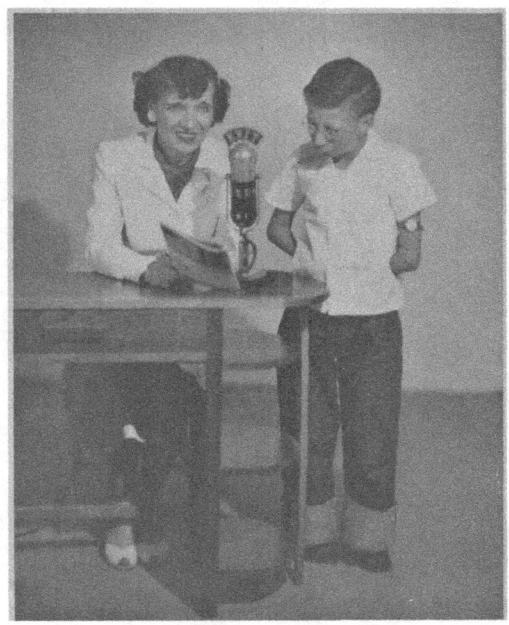

Gerry Wright and Shelby in 1951 at radio station KWFT looking at the People Today issue of April 25, 1951.

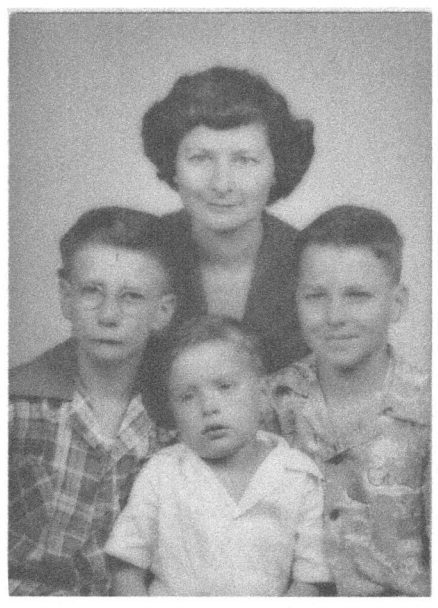

Shelby, Mother, David, and Ronnie on June 15, 1951

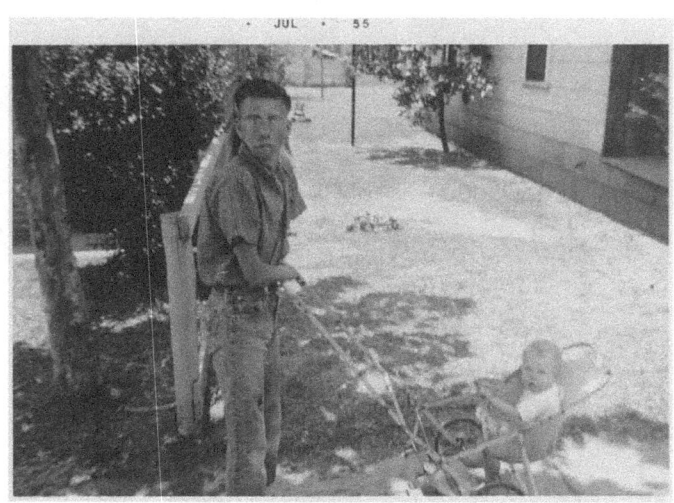

Shelby and Steve in front of Sonny's station and his home at 2803 York Street in July, 1955

AN INCREDIBLE BOY AND A REMARKABLE MAN

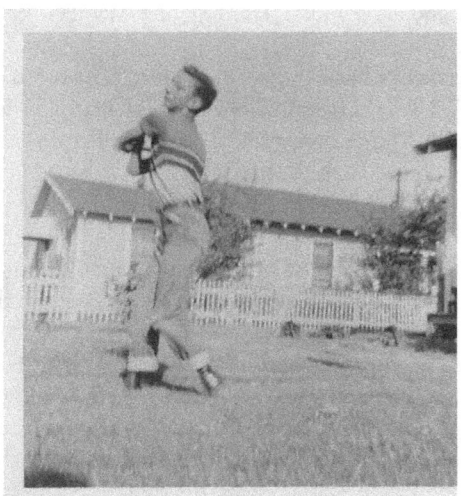

Shelby in his backyard in 1955

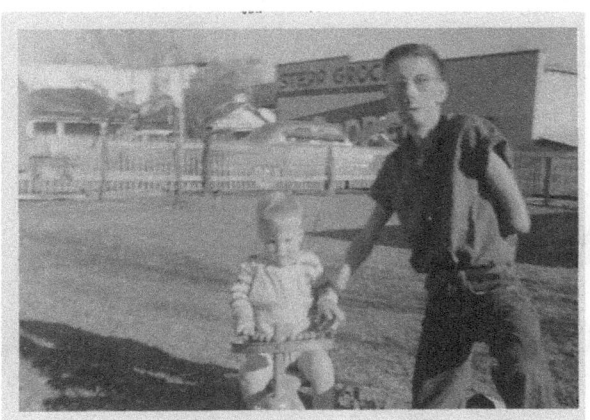

Shelby and Steve in 1956 with Stepp Grocery in
the background at 2604 Grant Street.

---

[1] Daddy always had five or six rattlesnake rattles inside his fiddle. Some fiddlers thought the rattles improved the sound. When I played Daddy's fiddle, it was a violin. I have two of those rattles as of July 30, 2020.

2. A series of books written from 1927 to 1951. We read the first book *Tower Treasure* (1927) and nine more. The last one was *The Wailing Siren Mystery* (1951).
3. Carl Schlemeyer quarterbacked the Odessa football team that lost to Houston Lamar in the 1953 Texas High School Football Championship game.
4. I have the slide rule, leather case, manual, and box. For no good reason, I cannot discard them, much less trash them.
5. Grandpa Ewing gave nicknames to all his children. He called Isaac "Son" and so did most of the family.
6. More will be told about the M & M Manufacturing Company in later chapters.
7. Uncle John and Aunt Velma called their son Sonny Boy and their daughter Sissy Girl.
8. It was 1873, the year that Colonel Robert M. Jones died. He was the owner of the Rose Hill plantation and a wealthy businessman. In 1946, Ron played with Norita Cody and four other children near the small graveyard. Also, Ron often went squirrel hunting in the heavily wooded Rose Hill when Ron made his summer visits with Uncle John and Aunt Velma from 1949 to 1953. Rose Hill was across the road from their home.

CHAPTER FIVE 5

Early Adult Years: Twenty to Twenty-Five (1956–61)

Shelby welcomed Rod and Ron home from college in late May 1956. They looked forward to being together on their church's softball team again. Rod and Ron had full-time summer jobs with the Texas Highway Department in Wichita Falls. They worked as swampers and roughnecks and loggers on a core-drilling rig. They liked working under driller Bill Lassiter and his assistant, Gordon Williams, and they learned the basics of drilling through marly clay and rock formations and recording the core samples. Their work would provide information for the highway engineers to determine where and at what depths to place the bridge pilings along the expressways and highways.

Shelby had not been able to find a job, so he visited with Darrell Spence, Butch, Uncle Sonny, Aunt Ruby, and Jim S. He also helped Mother take care of Stevie and worked some in Daddy's store by stocking shelves and sweeping.

Because Rod and Ron worked Monday through Friday and dated almost every night, they did not spend much time with Shelby that summer except the nights their church softball team played. Shelby began having more thoughts about what he was missing by not dating girls, but Mother did not encourage him to pursue such relationships.

Most of the players from the 1955 Highland Heights Baptist Church championship softball team played again in 1956. The team whizzed through the regular season undefeated. In the championship game, they were leading Southside Baptist 2 to 1 when a Texas National Guard jeep drove up. A master sergeant got out and walked to the plate umpire who called "time out." After a brief exchange, the umpire motioned for Rennie, their pitcher, to come to the plate. When the three finished a brief conversation, Rennie left with the master sergeant in the jeep. HHBC did not have another good pitcher, and they lost the game 2 to 4. They found out later that Rennie knew that he was required to attend an important National Guard meeting that night in preparation for summer camp. *Lesson learned by all, including Shelby, Rod, and Ron!*

The two Stepp families went to HHBC each Sunday. Shelby practiced playing his marimba every day, and he was still playing often in church services.

Mr. and Mrs. Lucas spent nearly all summer in Europe visiting servicemen that she had met at SAFB and touring popular places that she had been teaching about for many years in her geography and history classes. Ron wishes today that Shelby had kept the letters and postcards that she sent him during her travels.

She had accomplished so much in educating him during his ten years of public schooling, and she was rewarded with the joy and fulfillment of her contribution to his growing from childhood to adulthood.

That summer flew past, Sonny bought Rod a 1947 Chevrolet sedan, and Rod and Ron went back to college for their sophomore year. Shelby enrolled at Draughon's Business College in downtown Wichita Falls. He planned to earn a diploma in accounting and bookkeeping. Mother, Ruby, and Butch took Shelby to and from the college.

School year 1956–1957, Shelby studied basic business courses, which were not difficult for him. Having spent a lot of hours at a service station and a grocery store, he understood the basic operations of a business. His early courses were English, fundamental processes of business, and communications in a business environment.

AN INCREDIBLE BOY AND A REMARKABLE MAN

His three major adjustments in school were different teachers, a different student body, and a different location. Of course, his most challenging course was communications. As usual, he adapted to his new environment and made good grades and new friends.

Rod and Ron enjoyed military life in the A&M Corps, going to Aggie football games, and beginning long friendships. Their Aggies were ranked fifth in the nation in football at the end of the season with a record of nine wins, no losses, and one tie. They won the Southwest Conference championship. There were a handful of close, exciting games. One of those was a 19–13 victory over Shelby's Baylor Bears. The best was a 7–6 win over Texas Christian University in high wind, heavy rain, and lightning. The Aggies made two goal line stands late in the game. A 34–21 win over Texas in the final game made for a happy Thanksgiving. The girl from Wichita Falls whom Ron was going steady with came down for the game. She and Ron rode home with Aunt Ruby and Rod.

Shelby practiced playing his marimba almost every day, exercised and read the newspaper and listened to his radio daily, played his records and went to movies often, and attended church on Sunday and Wednesday. On many occasions, he visited Mrs. Lucas in her home, and they played marimba and piano duets at the local USO many times. She continued to encourage Shelby in his education and music activities.

Shelby attended the Coyote football team's home games and enjoyed watching them win their district without a defeat. Howard Franklin, Ron's friend who played on the Greyhound and Bronco baseball teams, was a star running back, passer, and punter. The Coyotes won their bi-district and regional playoff games, but they lost to Abilene 6–20 in the semifinal game. Shelby always enjoyed the marching bands too.

Mother began to often write in her letters that Daddy was getting disappointed about the slowdown of business in the store. People were shopping more often at the large supermarkets. Ron began to think about dropping out of school and working for one year to save enough to pay the $700 college expenses not covered by his scholarship.

In Major League Baseball (MLB), it was much the same old story. Another World Series pitting the New York Yankees against the Brooklyn Dodgers. Mickey Mantle completed the 1956 MLB regular season with a batting average of .353, 130 RBIs, and 52 homers to win the American League Triple Crown and most valuable player (MVP) awards. He also led the league in runs scored with 132 and slugging .705. Ron was very boastful to Shelby and Rod about those statistics and awards, but Brooklyn won games 1 and 2, and Shelby and Rod taunted Ron about those games. However, the Yankees pitchers threw five consecutive complete games (games 3–7) to cap off the comeback. No team had done that before, and none has done it since. Ron had bragging rights again.

The highlight of the series was *Don Larsen's perfect game* in game 5. Mantle saved Larsen's gem with a great running catch in left centerfield. He also homered in the 2–0 win. Ron was late for Shakespeare class because he listened to the game until the final out on his radio. When he got to class, several classmates whispered, "Did he get a no-hitter?"

Ron whispered back, "Yeah, and a perfect game too." Larsen was named the *Series MVP* for his historic pitching performance. The Dodgers scored nineteen runs in the first two games, but only six in the remaining five games including just one in the final three games. Over the years, Ron reminded Shelby, Rod, and Jim B. about the 1956 World Series from time to time.

Uncle Ike married an older widow who had two married daughters and an eleven-year-old son. She worked at SAFB and attended Draughon's Business College. They lived on Grant Street about eight blocks from the L. R. Stepp's house. Shelby began to visit often with Ike, Imogene, her son Russell, and Pam.

On several Sundays, Shelby played his marimba at the SAFB Service Club. Most of the airmen who attended were those who could not get a pass to leave the base. At that time, Shelby had three connections with Aunt Imogene: Draughon's, SAFB, and Ike. They had good times together for many years until Imogene died in early 1994.

AN INCREDIBLE BOY AND A REMARKABLE MAN

Christmas 1956, the seven Stepp boys observed their early Christmas morning tradition. Their relationships were still strong, but their times together were less than before because Rod and Ron dated almost every night and helped their dads at the station and the store on most days during the holidays. Mother was also working often at the store, which required Shelby to babysit Stevie and supervise David. Their families enjoyed going to church together for two Sundays.

Ron talked Daddy into driving down to Archer City to look at the new 1957 Chevrolet Bel Airs. He drove one that was Sierra Gold (bottom) and Adobe Beige (top), liked it, made a deal, and bought it. He drove it home and told Mother that it was the car he had always wanted. Cousin Ernest Johnston, who worked at the Cadillac and Pontiac dealership in Wichita Falls, told Daddy that he paid about $2,000 less than what it would have cost in Wichita Falls. Our family really liked that car. When Mother would ask Stevie, "Whose car is that?" he would say "Bub Bub." He called Ron "Bub Bub" in his early years.

Before going back to school, Ron gave an engagement ring to his fiancée, and they planned to get married after his junior year. She also planned to get employment in Wichita Falls after high school graduation in May 1957 and after they got married to get employment in Bryan and College Station while Ron finished his double degree requirements.

Back in school after the holidays, Shelby worked hard on his schoolwork and made good grades in the first semester. Rod and Ron did the same, and in early February, they completed the first semester and headed home for about five days. Ron discovered that Daddy had sold the new car a few days before. Daddy could not stand to owe anyone much money for a long period. Ron joined Mother, Shelby, and David in their disappointment about losing their dream car.

Shelby completed his first year at Draughon's Business College with good grades. Rod and Ron completed their second year at Texas A&M with good grades. Rod got a summer job with Shell Oil working on a seismic crew in East Texas. Shelby helped care for Stevie and helped with stocking and sweeping at the store. Shelby continued to play his marimba in church services often.

Ron worked at the Texas Highway Department in Wichita Falls again. Most of the summer, he was on a bridge survey crew on three new expressways being constructed. The route of one of the expressways eliminated the house of Uncle Tommy and Aunt Nila Ewing and their Brook Avenue Baptist Church building. Ron told the family about surveying on the former Ewing property where a bridge would be constructed.

Ron joined Downtown Baptist Church (DBC), formerly Brook Avenue Baptist Church, which had relocated in the former building of Lamar Baptist Church. He wanted to play on a softball team that could go to the state playoffs. He went to Sunday school and morning and evening worship services every Sunday. For the first time, Shelby would be the batboy for one of Ron's opponents.

When DBC played HHBC, Ron hit two homers and DBC beat HHBC soundly. Ron told Shelby after the game that he did not feel good about the game because he had more close friends on the HHBC team than on the DBC team. Shelby did not have much to say about it. DBC won the church league and went to the church state softball playoffs in Brownwood. They won the first two games, but they lost in the semifinals. Tyler Owen, a legendary softball pitcher in his prime, was the ace pitcher for DBC.

All summer Ron worked forty hours a week, played two softball games each week, and dated most nights. He did not spend much time with Shelby. Although Shelby did not work much and did not date any, he was always on the go. He attended church every Sunday morning and night and Wednesday night, went to movies once or twice each week with Butch and others, was batboy for the HHBC men's softball team, often played ball in his backyard with four or five boys including Jim S., David, and Joe, and helped boys pass the Morse code requirements for earning their first-class Scout Badge. He played his marimba every day.

In September 1957, Shelby began his first business accounting course, a second course in communications, and a basic course in business management. The accounting and management courses were almost totally new to him and were challenging.

Rod and Ron were each taking several courses, which included a three-hour laboratory period. Those labs increased their hours in class significantly. Ron was taking eighteen to twenty-one hours each semester, which were too many for difficult subjects. He began to struggle with his studies.

In the Cadet Corps, Ron was a technical sergeant on the First Battalion staff of the Second Regiment, which was a high position in the Corps of Cadets for a junior. He was selected to serve as co-editor of the sports section of the Aggieland yearbook staff.

Rod was selected to join the Ross Volunteers, which was an elite group. Rod was also selected to serve as co-editor of the organizations section of the Aggieland yearbook staff.

In early September, Asiatic flu broke out among the students and quickly filled the local hospitals. Those in the corps who did not have the flu carried food from the two campus mess halls and distributed medications to the many sick students in their beds in the dorms. Rod delivered medications while Ron distributed food. They did that all week.

After classes on Saturday morning, Ron rode to Lubbock with four Aggies to attend the Texas Tech football game that night. He began to feel sick during the trip. They arrived in Lubbock, and Ron went to the game with his fiancée who had driven from Wichita Falls with several other girls who dated Aggies.

The Aggies won the game 21–0 without John David Crow and Loyd Taylor, but Ron was quite ill by the end of the game. He went to a party with his fiancée and five or six of his Aggie buddies, but on arrival, his flu symptoms had peaked. Ron did not drink alcoholic beverages, but one of his buddies handed him a glass half full of bourbon and told him to drink all of it without stopping, and it would help him sleep despite the flu. He drank it and then went to lie down on a quilt on a bedroom floor while the others partied. He was told the next morning that he had slept like a baby. It was mostly a lost weekend for Ron and his fiancée.

The Aggies won their first eight games, including a 14 to 0 win over Shelby's Baylor Bears, and were ranked number 1 in the nation. Five days before game 9 against Rice, word leaked out on campus that Coach Paul "Bear" Bryant was leaving A&M after the football season to coach his alma mater, the University of Alabama. All week, the football team and student body got more and more disheartened about losing Coach Bryant.

Rice outscored Texas A&M 7 to 6, then Texas outscored the Aggies 9 to 7, and in the Gator Bowl Tennessee outscored them 3 to 0. The Aggies had a lot of turnovers in all three games. John David Crow and Charlie Krueger made All-American first team, and Crow was awarded the Heisman Trophy. Shelby wrote Ron a "mean" letter[1] immediately after the A&M versus Rice game.

Shelby went to most of the Coyotes football home games, and they had a good season. They won their district and then won the bi-district game, but they lost to Dallas Highland Park in the quarterfinal game. Highland Park went on to win the state championship.

In Major League Baseball the Milwaukee Braves won the National League pennant. Shelby's Dodgers finished in third place. That was the last of the Brooklyn Dodgers. They moved to Los Angeles after the season ended, but Shelby and Rod continued to be avid Dodger fans. The New York Yankees won the American League again but lost to the Braves in the seventh game of the World Series. Braves' pitcher Lew Burdette pitched three outstanding games and won all of them and was voted most valuable player.

Lloyd Stone, one of Ron's best buddies in junior high and high school and a friend to Shelby, had completed two years of college at Tarleton State, which was in the Texas A&M System. For two seasons on a baseball scholarship, he had been their starting catcher. He enrolled at A&M in September 1957 on a baseball scholarship. He and Ron got to see each other often.

On Christmas Day 1957, the seven Stepp boys kept their early Christmas morning tradition intact. Rod, Butch, and Jim woke up about 5:00 a.m. and opened their gifts with their mom and dad. Then they walked two blocks to the other Stepp house and woke Shelby, Ron, David, and Stevie. They showed them some of their gifts and told them about the others. Then they watched as Shelby and his brothers opened their gifts. Shelby got a new radio. Steve got mostly toys. Again, clothes were popular gifts. They visited a while and played with David's toys and helped Stevie play with his toys.

The Stepp families enjoyed going to church together for two Sundays. Rod and Ron dated almost every night and helped their dads at the station and the store on most days. Shelby, Ron, and David watched the Rose Bowl Parade and several bowl games. Shelby never missed the Rose Bowl Parade and always watched the four major bowl games and some of the other bowl games. Shelby continued to babysit Stevie and watch David when Mother worked in the store.

Not all of Shelby's childcare was fun and games. Following are selected entries in his 1958 diary.

> This evening I almost had a nervous breakdown because of David's continuous tantalization of Steve. When Mother came home, I immediately got out of the house and went to the store. (January 3, 1958)

But Shelby had fun with family and friends.

> This afternoon I witnessed test firings of a rocket car performed by Butch and his buddies Nelson and Bryan on the parking lot next door to our house. (Saturday, January 4)

After the holiday break from school, Shelby, Rod, and Ron resumed their college work. Shelby questioned the course of study he had selected.

> I returned to school today. I was rather worried because of hearing a decision pertinent to whether I should continue taking bookkeeping. (January 6)

This afternoon I watched the very exciting Senior Bowl gridiron classic matching the North's Collegian All Stars and the South's. The Northerners squeezed by 15-13. (January 11)

When I went to get me a soda pop this afternoon, I was thrilled to walk in the mud. (January 14) [The weather had been very dry.]

This evening one of my former classmates at Austin Elementary, H. D. Smith, came to visit me. He and I carried on conversations mostly pertaining to females. He likes girls. (January 17)

I am standing here by the dresser looking at a handsome-looking brute in the mirror. His name is Shelby Stepp. (January 21)

Tonight I studied my bookkeeping through the waning hours of the night. Results: Nothing accomplished. (January 23)

Tonight I listened to a thrilling basketball game between the Coyotes and Arlington. The Pack kept their district record clean winning 49-46. (January 24)

Ronnie came home from Texas A&M for a five-day semester holiday. I was exceedingly delighted to see him back home. (January 25)

If space would allow me to write everything, I'd like to say about what happened at HHBC tonight, just let me say there was a spiritual revival there. (Sunday, January 26)

I'm sitting here in my bed looking at the picture of Ronnie's fiancée, thinking how lucky I'll be to have a beautiful sister-in-law someday. (January 27)

AN INCREDIBLE BOY AND A REMARKABLE MAN

Shelby never revealed any hope of having his own beautiful fiancée.

> I sat up until 12:00 tonight listening to the rock and roll music. Boy, I just dig that sweet music. (January 28)

Is "rock and roll" really "sweet" music? I guess it is all in the ears of the listener.

The night before going back to college, Ron told his fiancée that he wanted to wait until after his senior year at A&M to get married. She got upset with him. Ron did not blame her, but he was not going to be ready to marry until he improved his financial status and made good grades. About a week later, Mother told Ron in a letter that his ex-fiancée had returned the engagement ring to her.

When Ron got back to Texas A&M to finish the second semester of his junior year, he talked to the dean of the engineering college and told him that he wanted to change his major to prepare to teach high school math and history and coach baseball. Dean Calhoun talked Ron into adopting a bachelor of science degree in civil engineering, which would give him enough additional math courses to teach math. Ron changed his degree plan.

Lloyd tried to talk Ron into going out for the Aggie baseball team, but Ron did not think he should because of struggling to make good grades. When Ron registered for his second semester courses, he knowingly signed up for an engineering course, which required a prerequisite course that he had not taken. That ended up being a big problem for him.

Mother wrote Ron often, and in one of her letters, she told him that his ex-fiancée was engaged to be married in June.

More entries from Shelby's 1958 diary follow.

> I've just arrived home from riding around with Ruby and J. D. [Aunt Ruby's boyfriend after Uncle Sonny and Aunt Ruby had separated].

We had a grand time chatting and telling jokes. (February 1)

I didn't do anything but work on bookkeeping during the entire afternoon. I'm stuck on a problem that's got me down. (Sunday, February 2)

I attended Prayer Meeting tonight and they continue to be good, old spiritual gatherings. (February 5)

I went to visit the Troop 6 weekly (scout) meeting tonight and see Mr. Nathan Gould the scoutmaster, who helped me accomplish so much in scouting. (February 6)

I had a very busy day assisting two boys pass the Morse code requirements. Only one of them passed. (February 8)

This evening I attended the 15th Troop 6 Annual Court of Honor. I was indeed proud and honored to be certified as assistant scoutmaster of code. (February 9)

This afternoon I went to Hawkins Variety Store and bought a Valentine box of candy for my mother. (February 13)

I went over to the Olympic Food Store and drank a bottle of Dr. Pepper. I like to patronize them because they are friendly. (Sunday, February 16)

Wow! I just got through listening to the Coyotes nip Denton in a double overtime basketball game 41-39 to take the lead in a best of three playoff series. (February 19)

AN INCREDIBLE BOY AND A REMARKABLE MAN

The Coyotes lost to Denton in the second game, but they beat Denton in the third game to advance to bi-district playoffs against Lufkin.

> This afternoon I went to a movie at the new Parker Square Theater to see my favorite actor Rock Hudson in "The Tarnished Angels." (February 23)
>
> Tonight I listened to the Coyotes win a close game in bi-district against Lufkin. The final was 50-46. (February 24)
>
> I am very upset at the present moment because the Coyotes were eliminated in a 4-A Regional game by Dallas Woodrow Wilson. (February 28)
>
> I went to Prayer Meeting tonight and during the session of prayer I went down to the altar with a group of men and knelt in prayer. (March 5)
>
> I listened to the last portion of the Red River Boxing Tournament tonight on KTRN radio. Jack Britton was the blow-by-blow announcer. (March 7)
>
> I went out to the store not only to drink a Dr. Pepper but to visit with Uncle Sonny who has moved back from Fort Worth. (March 8) [Sonny would soon move back to Fort Worth to live there for the rest of his life.]
>
> I had the house to myself most of the afternoon while Daddy and Mother, David and Steve went in our new hot rod [a much-used 1950 Ford]. I really enjoyed myself during this time. (Sunday, March 9)
>
> This afternoon as soon as I got home from school, I shaved off the fuzzy whiskers. It was the first time I had shaved in 11 days. (March 13)

I helped a boy by the name of Glen McShan pass the Morse code test. Even though it kept me from watching television I enjoyed it. (March 15) [Glen later became one of David's best buddies.]

I practiced on my marimba on two songs that I am to play for the Texas A&M Mothers Club. (March 18)

I continued my music practice after school this afternoon. I practiced for two hours and ten minutes. (Wednesday, March 19)

This afternoon I played two marimba solos for the Texas A&M Mothers Club. (March 21)

This evening I watched a good play "The Hallmark Hall of Fame" on television. The title of the play was "Little Moon of Alban." (March 24)

I completed the "Public Accounting" book this afternoon. Tomorrow I will begin the "Automobile" book. (March 26)

Today was a great inspirational time at our church as we heard two great sermons. Our Pastor Reverend Newberry preached in the morning and Gerald Phillips[2] preached in the evening and dedicated his life to the ministry. (Sunday, March 30)

Tonight I watched my favorite TV program "Suspicion."[3] (March 31)

Today there was an historical event in Wichita Falls as a small tornado struck the outskirts of the city.[4] (April 2)

Today I became ill in school just after eating lunch. After school I came home and laid down. (April 7)

Happy Birthday to poor old healthless me. Even though it seems a hopeless case to get well,

AN INCREDIBLE BOY AND A REMARKABLE MAN

> I still have enough strength to observe my 22nd birthday. (April 8)
>
> Tonight I sing He Leadeth Me which seems proper for Jesus really guided a sick man to church tonight. (Wednesday, April 9)
>
> Behold I bring you "Good Tidings." I am about to overcome this long and sickening illness. (April 10)
>
> Hurrah! Great days are here again! I am now a man of health again. (April 11)

About this time, Uncle Louis and Uncle Sonny each came up with $5,000 to buy the bankrupt sheet metal pipe and duct workshop where Sonny had been working in Fort Worth. They named the company M&M Manufacturing Company (both their middle initials were M). Louis continued to work at Barrow Grace Buick.

> Tonight was the climax of a successful revival. Seventeen of those 21 who made professions of faith were baptized. (Sunday, April 20)
>
> I just got through viewing the late movie called "The 3 Godfathers." The featured stars were John Wayne and Harry Carey, Jr. (April 28)
>
> I just got through eating a two-hour supper. It certainly was delicious. For dessert I had German chocolate cake. (April 29)
>
> During the Prayer Meeting at our church, the people made plans to have a reception for our new education director Malcolm Sample. (Wednesday, April 30)
>
> I have been working on bookkeeping preparing a trial balance sheet.[5] (May 1)

Shelby completed his second year at Draughon's Business College with good grades, but he lacked meaningful things to do with much of his time. Sonny leased his service station to a neighbor and moved to Fort Worth. Earlier he and Ruby had separated, and he had been living in the station for months. In Fort Worth, he went to work in a sheet metal pipe and duct workshop owned by a friend from his Hugo days. Shelby was heartbroken over the separation and Sonny not being around to visit. The lives of Shelby, Rod, and Ron were beginning to be more challenging in multiple dimensions.

>I spent my first day of school vacation by lounging around, reading, and listening to my radio. Ironically, I wish I were in school. (Friday, May 9)
>
>Tonight J. D., David, and I went to the movies at Grant St. Drive-In. Two of the features were good, but the third one was boring. (May 10)
>
>He did it! He did it! Stan Musial got his 3000th hit—a double. And I heard it on my radio. (May 13)
>
>I didn't do much of anything but lay around and wished I was back in school. (May 15)
>
>I am filled with enthusiasm tonight because tomorrow at 4:00 AM I am going to Fort Worth to see Uncle John. (May 23)
>
>I have just arrived back from Fort Worth. The travel time was 2 hours and 30 minutes. I really had a splendid time. (Saturday, May 24)
>
>Dad put in our air conditioner this afternoon. Having had such sweltering weather lately I sighed with relief. (May 25)
>
>Tonight I watched two of my four favorite TV western shows, "Wyatt Earp" and "Tales of Wells Fargo." (May 26)
>
>Tonight I asked Uncle Louis to come over and when he came I asked him for a job where he works. He said there was no chance because the business is taking its lumps. (May 29) [Louis

was the service manager at Barrow Grace Buick dealership. He resigned six months later because business was not good under the new ownership.]

This morning I received a telephone call from a Captain in the National Guard Unit indicating my name was presented to him as a draftee. Because of my physical defects I could not answer the call. (May 30) [He could not answer the "call to duty."]

Tonight after taking a good bath, I had my favorite dessert German Chocolate Cake with ice cream for topping. M-m-m-m. (May 31)

Rod and Ron finished their junior year at Texas A&M. Rod's grades continued to be good. Aggie students in geological engineering degree plans were required to take a six-week geology field trip course in the summer after their junior year. Those in the Corps of Cadets were also required to take a six-week ROTC training course at a US military base in the summer after their junior year.

Rod chose to go to the geology field trip first and go to Fort Sill the following summer. During the first half of summer, he took two courses at Texas A&M and worked as editor of the *Aggieland* yearbook for 1958 to get it published on schedule. The *Aggieland* editor had gotten married and asked Rod to replace him and finish the yearbook. Rod spent the second half of summer at geology camp in Junction and Big Bend.

Ron chose to work for the Texas Highway Department the first half of summer as a paving inspector, play softball for Downtown Baptist, and then go to Fort Sill, Oklahoma, for the required six-week ROTC training.

Butch graduated from Wichita Falls Senior High and moved to Fort Worth to work with his daddy. Jim finished ninth grade at Zundy junior high, and David completed sixth grade at Sam Houston grade school. Jim Booher graduated from Texas Tech with a bachelor of science in architecture.

Shelby worked in the store, helped care for almost three-year-old Stevie, but did not hang out at the station because Uncle Sonny and Butch were gone.

The following are more entries from Shelby's diary for 1958.

> Today my daddy and I watched the last four innings of a game between the Cincinnati Reds and Philadelphia. This was the first game televised on Sunday. (Sunday, June 1)
>
> Today Lloyd Stone, a longtime buddy of Ronnie, came over this evening to go with the latter to a softball game. [Shelby would not miss prayer meeting.] (June 4)
>
> This morning I had a wonderful time playing baseball with David and his gang. I was surprised that I could still powder the ball. I got 7 hits in 10 at bats. (June 5)
>
> I watched a baseball game between Cleveland and New York on TV this afternoon. The Yankees won 6-3. (June 7)
>
> I watched the second game of the series between Cleveland and New York. This time the tables were reversed as the Indians won easily 14-1. (Sunday, June 8)
>
> Tonight for the first time in many moons, I saw my cousin Jerry Ewing. He had brought Ronnie home to get ready for a ball game. (June 9)
>
> This afternoon I received shocking news that Joyce Spence, my former classmate in grade school died this morning in a hospital in Dallas. She had an operation yesterday to correct a heart ailment. (Wednesday, June 11)
>
> This morning I had another one of those big surprises, but this time a wonderful one.

> Darrell came to see me. He had come home from Lexington (Texas). (June 13)
>
> I sat up 'til midnight tonight listening to some music on the radio. I had some company of chiggers biting all over me while I was listening. (June 17)
>
> After prayer meeting, I went to the movies with Ruby and J. D. out at the Seymour Drive-In. The features were "The Big Land" and "Darby's Rangers." I had seen the former before. (June 18)
>
> Tonight Darrell and I went to a BTU party at Barbara King's home. We had to walk all the way to 3009 Lawrence, but we got a ride home. (June 19) [BTU was Baptist Training Union.]
>
> This afternoon Bill Stallcup came over to visit with me for four hours. I enjoyed every minute conversing with him. He asked me if I would like to go with him to a Youth Rally. I consented. (June 20) [Bill was confined to a wheelchair, but he was very active in Christian evangelism.]
>
> Tonight my mother is walking around here with her eyes half-closed. She said she is going to hit the sack after she gives me a bath. (June 21)

Ron and Rennie Havens went to Ron's ex-fiancée's wedding. It turned a few heads when Ron walked into the church. During the wedding ceremony, Ron felt strongly that he was not ready to get married and wished the best for her marriage.

> This afternoon I received a phone call from Mrs. Lucas requesting that I bring my marimba over to her home so we could practice. She said that we were booked for the USO next Saturday. (June 23)
>
> I went over to Mrs. Lucas' to practice some more this afternoon. We began to work on a cou-

ple of new songs, "I'll String Along with You" and "Beautiful Ohio." She let me take the former music home to practice on it. (June 24)

This evening I went over to Mrs. Lucas' at her request to play some music for Dr. George R. Davis and his wife. (Wednesday, June 25)

This morning Dennis and Roger came over to mow our lawn. Afterwards we spent the rest of the morning talking and tussling around. (June 26) [Dennis and Roger Mansell were cousins on the Ewing side. They were sons of Aunt Almeda.]

This evening I had the privilege of playing two marimba solos, "Holy City" and "My God and I," for the Union Services at First Christian Church. (Sunday, June 29)

I went to the Texas Employment Commission to enter my application for a bookkeeping job. They said they would notify me. (June 30)

Today I started my first day helping Mother run the store because Daddy began working part-time at his new job. (July 1) [Daddy worked part-time at Midwestern University as a carpenter and painter.]

In 2020, Steve wrote this memory of his relationship with Shelby in mid-1958:

> I don't really remember what my thoughts were of Shelby's physical challenges when I was almost four years old. He had mastered so much by the time I came along. Dad went to work for Midwestern University as a carpenter and Mom ran the store, so Shelby would have to watch after me sometimes. I remember sitting on the front porch at 2803 York St. with Shelby and we would

AN INCREDIBLE BOY AND A REMARKABLE MAN

have a Dr. Pepper and a Mr. Goodbar at least once a week. Boy, that was delicious. It seemed that Shelby always had his transistor radio with him wherever he went, listening to music or preferably a baseball or basketball game, if he could find one. To tell you the truth, I think Shelby kept up with all sports. He was definitely a diehard Dodgers fan.

I am really pooped tonight after working all day at the store. Worst of all, my legs are aching. (July 2)

This evening I had the privilege of attending a Brotherhood meeting out at Lake Wichita Baptist Church with Bill Stallcup. I really enjoyed it. (July 3)

This evening Darrell and I went to see the Academy Award winning movie, "Sayonara." It was the best romantic movie I've ever seen. (July 4)

Tonight I went out again. This time my accompanist, Mrs. Thelma Lucas and I performed a 45-minute music program at the USO. I was really received well by the crowd. (July 5)

Tonight I went to another one of those 1950s Academy Award winning movies, "Peyton Place." Unfortunately, I missed the last part because I was snoozing. (July 7)

After prayer meeting I went over to Rex Moody's to chat a little while. We really had a wonderful time telling jokes and beating on each other. (Wednesday, July 9)

Ronnie came from Fort Sill for the weekend. He is going to stay with Rennie Havens while he's here. (July 11)

Today the one-week Youth Revival started at our church. Providing the dynamic sermons and exquisite singing are Lloyd Pierson and Wayne Monroe respectively. (Sunday, July 13)

Tonight I went to a Baptist Associational Brotherhood meeting in Electra with a couple of guys from Lake Wichita Baptist. (July 14)

Again I hanged out. This time it was at a dance hall. The reason for my presence was to play some marimba solos. (July 15) [I wish Shelby had written the names of the songs he played. Knowing him, they may have included hymns.]

Well, I was finally overcome by the wrath of God because I had no excuse not to be in church! So this time I went. (July 16)

Tonight I heard a wonderful sermon by Lloyd called "The Fourth Man." It was about Shadrach, Meshach, and Abednego being cast into fire. (July 17)

Please believe what I have to say. I didn't get to go to church tonight because I had to babysit. I'll go tomorrow. (July 18)

Tonight I went to church again. See, I told you I would. (July 19)

Tonight I played a couple of special marimba solos during the prelude and again during the offertory at our church. (Sunday, July 20)

This evening I worked out at the store until closing time [usually 9:00 p.m.]. (July 26)

I went over to Mrs. Lucas' this afternoon to play some music for her guest. The latter was a young airman. (Sunday, July 27)

Wow! The humidity is terrific today! I'm sure glad I get to work in a good air-conditioned place like the store. (July 30)

Tonight David had Larry Slack to spend the night with him. They almost drove us insane because they cut-up and giggled nearly all night long. (July 31)

Today Ronnie came home to stay following his completion of six weeks ROTC training at Fort Sill. (August 1)

Today I just laid around the house—which is very unusual for me to do—Ha Ha! I watched TV. (August 2)

This morning I had a visitor come to see me at the store. We had a swell time teasing about our respective baseball clubs. (August 5)

Tonight I did something that I very seldom do. I missed prayer meeting and my only excuse was that I wanted to work at the store. (August 6)

I received a phone call from Bill Stallcup reminding me about the watermelon party at his church. He asked if I still wanted to go and I told him I had to work. (August 7)

This morning I had another visit from my good friend. He asked me if I would like to go see him and his team play. I said that I would think about it. (August 11)

I have been a sick man today with the flu. Because of this terrible illness, I had to be confined to the bed all day. (Tuesday, August 12)

Despite my weakness from the flu, I worked at the store today to make up for yesterday's absence. (August 13)

Tonight I went to the ball game with my friend. What a night it was. His team got beat, I had a headache, and his car had a flat and he had no spare. (August 14)

Tonight I watched the College Football All Stars play the Pro Champion Detroit Lions. The

College All Stars really showed them up by winning 32–14. (August 15)

This afternoon I went out in the backyard and pitched a tennis ball against the store building to get myself in shape. (Sunday, August 17)

Once again I had another visit from my friend at the store. We talked about how the world championship fight between Patterson and Harris would come out. I picked Patterson. (August 18) [Patterson won by a KO in the thirteenth round.]

At noon I watched a romantic movie, In the Meantime, Darling. I really enjoyed the hugging and kissing that went on in it. (August 19) [Shelby had never kissed anyone. Without lips and related muscles, he could not perform a normal kiss.]

Hum-m-m excuse me for my expression. I'm very sleepy tonight. Boy, I got to go to bed pronto, dagnabbit. (August 25)

I worked out at the store a little longer than usual tonight. When I went home to eat, the food sure tasted delicious after a long day's work. (August 26)

Tonight I went over to Mrs. Lucas' to play some marimba solos for her guest from Saudi Arabia. (August 27) [The guest was probably a Saudi military pilot training at SAFB.]

I was really angered this evening at Ronnie because he prevented Mother from punishing Steve when the latter really needed it too. I really wanted to tear into him regardless of his size. (Thursday, August 28) [Ron was not aware that he upset Shelby.]

> I've just come out from the store after a long day's work. It was wonderful to get back to labor. (September 2)

Back in school in September 1958, Shelby continued at Draughon's Business College with courses in accounting and bookkeeping and business law. He did well the first semester. Rod was selected to serve on the First Battalion staff of the Second Regiment as a major and continued to serve on the Ross Volunteers and was editor of the Aggieland yearbook staff. He continued his courses for a geological engineering degree and made good grades the first semester. Ron was selected to serve as a major on the Second Regimental staff and was majoring in civil engineering. Jim began the ninth grade at Zundy, and David started the sixth grade.

> I discovered something today which practically knocked me for a loop. As the school kids came by our store to buy "junk," I was greatly overcome by school fever as I saw their books. (September 5)
>
> Tonight I went over to Darrell's house to watch the Miss America Pageant. Wow!. Those dames were beautiful and attractive. (September 6)
>
> I have just completed studying the fourth chapter of Auditing. (September 11)
>
> Tonight I heard a good sermon given by Rev. Newberry on "Christian Faith." He based his message on David and Goliath. (Sunday, September 14)
>
> I have just stopped working on a problem in Auditing. Unfortunately, with such stupidity, I could not work it. (September 15)
>
> Today our church had a semi-reawakening. Rev. Newberry repented for not executing duties of a pastor, and some church officers pub-

licly promised they would do better. (Sunday, September 21)

After I got home from school I went out to the store and helped my mother. (September 25) [This was Stevie's fourth birthday.]

This afternoon prior to beginning my studies I wrote a letter to Aunt Velma who resides in Hugo, Oklahoma. (Sunday, September 28)

I am sitting here thinking about the time that I was double-crossed by a girl whom I really cared about when we were in school together. (September 30)

I was highly enthused today after hearing that Milwaukee took the first game of the World Series against the New York Yankees, 4-3. (October 1)

Tonight I saw a very good dramatic play called "Days of Wine and Roses" on Playhouse 90. It was about a couple who fought alcoholism. (October 2)

This afternoon I watched the third game of the World Series on TV. Unfortunately, the Yankees won 4-0, but they still trail 1-2. (October 4)

Tonight I attended one of the best Fellowship meetings our church has ever held. A hilarious play was performed and wonderful games were played. (Sunday, October 5)

From the time I got home from school to now, I've been studying "Inventories" in Chapter 9 of Auditing. (October 6)

Tonight for the first time this season I went to watch a Coyotes football game.

They tangled the Vernon Lions by a score of 47-0. (October 10)

I attended the first of four nights of a study course of Baptist History. (Monday, October 13)

I have just completed a letter to Aunt Velma. As I glance at the clock, it shows that I am late for bed. (October 16)

Tonight I listened to a very exciting and well fought football game between the Coyotes and Odessa High. We won 20-6. (October 17)

This afternoon my daddy and I watched a professional football game between the Chicago Bears and the Los Angeles Rams. The Bears won 31-10. (October 19)

Tonight I am having a good time working some Auditing problems in Chapter 11 because you know what? This is the easiest I've had thus far this year! (October 21)

I'm still having an easy time with my Auditing course. (October 22)

I have just come home from watching one of Texas' top Class 4A football games between the Coyotes and Corpus Christi. The Coyotes won 34-0. (October 24)

I've just completed my studies. Unfortunately, I collided with quite a problem. (October 27)

This evening I went to see the Coyote football team play their district opener against the Irving Tigers. The Pack won 58-22. (October 31)

This morning I got lonesome sitting during the Church Services because my buddies Butch and Nelson were not there. (Sunday, November 2)

I've just got through hearing wonderful news that the Democrats had regained Congress in the election. (November 4)

I am very sick tonight with what is apparently a case of virus. Mother and David have it too. (November 6)

Tonight I listened to the Coyote—Arlington football game. The Coyotes continued to roll with a 24-0 victory. (November 7)

This afternoon Mrs. Lucas and I went to the USO to play during the Vesper Services. (Sunday, November 9)

I went over to Mrs. Lucas' tonight to practice on some music that we plan to play for the Fun Night at Austin Grade School on Friday night. (November 10)

I've just completed studying about the Audit Report in Chapter 17 of Auditing. (November 13)

Tonight I represented my old pride and joy Room 7 at Austin Grade School by playing my marimba at the annual Fun Night. (November 14)

Today I watched a Southwest Conference football game between TCU and Texas. The Horned Frogs won 21-7. (November 15)

This afternoon Mrs. Lucas and I went to the USO to play for the Vesper Services. We accompanied the congregational singing and then played some special music. (Sun. November 16)

I've just completed my nightly studies. This stuff certainly does wear me out. (November 17)

Cold wintry weather prevailed throughout the day. This type of weather pleases me exceedingly. (November 18)

I stayed out at the store to help my dad. (November 21)

After coming home from drinking a pop at the store, I studied the Auditing book for a couple of hours. (Saturday, November 22)

AN INCREDIBLE BOY AND A REMARKABLE MAN

About this time, Uncle Louis quit his job at Barrow Grace Buick and went to work for M&M. He did not want to leave Wichita Falls, so he worked in Fort Worth Tuesday through Friday each week, and he hauled products home and sold them out of his two-car garage on Saturday and Monday of each week. On weekdays, Aunt Lydia sold products in Wichita Falls. This schedule continued for about two years.

> This morning our church had its Annual Pledge March. By department and class each class member placed their tithing pledge cards on the altar. (Sunday, November 23)
>
> This afternoon Butch brought his portable TV to let me watch the football games. He is working on our TV. (November 27)
>
> Tonight in church we watched a slide presentation about foreign missions and the Lottie Moon Christmas offering. (Sunday, November 30)
>
> This evening Butch brought our TV back after working on it for a week. He did a fine job. (December 1)
>
> I sat up 'til 11:00 working on a problem in Auditing. I'm a little weary. (December 4)
>
> Tonight I watched a brawling 15 round welterweight championship fight between Virgil Akins and Don Jordan. The latter won the fight and the title. (December 5)
>
> This afternoon I heard the Coyotes trounce Abilene, the state's top-rated team, in the quarterfinals 34-6. It was the biggest upset of the year. (December 6)
>
> This morning I completed another problem in Chapter 18 of Auditing. Only two more problems remain to be worked. (Monday, December 8)

I was a little frightened today when Butch was later than usual to pick me up at school. He's forgotten to pick me up several times this year. (December 9)

This afternoon I listened to the Class 4A Semifinal game in which the Coyotes edged Dallas Highland Park 22-14. The Pack advances to the state championship game next week. (December 13)

This morning I contributed $5 to the Lottie Moon Christmas Offering. (Sunday, December 14)

Tonight Mother and I went downtown to do our Christmas shopping. I spent $8 to get gifts for David, Steve, and Darrell. (December 16)

Due to a party which was hosted by my mother for her Sunday School teachers, I went to Parker Square English Pharmacy until the party was over. (December 18) [Mother was a department director as well as a teacher in Sunday school.]

I sat up until 11:45 addressing Christmas cards. Believe you me I am tired. (December 19)

Shelby went to the Coyotes football home games all season, and with his fan support, they played in the state championship game in Austin on December 20. Rod and Ron drove over to Austin to watch the game on their way home for the Christmas holidays. The Coyotes beat Pasadena 48 to 6. The Aggie football team without Coach Bryant won four games and lost six, but they beat Shelby's Baylor Bears for the fourth year in a row, 33 to 27.

Ronnie has just come in to stay during his two weeks Christmas vacation. (December 20)

[Shelby did not mention that today was Daddy's fifty-fourth birthday.]

Today a special Christmas program was presented at our church by the four choirs. It was indeed an excellent service. (Sunday, December 21)

I babysat Steve today. To keep myself from going into hysterics, I worked on bookkeeping. (December 22)

As I write this entry, I am sitting at my new desk. I was surprised to hear tonight that this is my Christmas present from my parents. Although I was glad to get it, I was very disappointed to have my Christmas a day earlier than everybody else. (December 24)

Christmas morning 1958, the seven Stepp boys kept their tradition in good order. Everyone got clothes, Shelby showed everyone his desk, and Stevie got some toys.

This evening I watched the 34th Annual Shrine Bowl game pitting West vs. East. It was a well fought game with the East winning 26-14. (December 27)

Tonight our church held a special program which is called "Student Night" which honors the members attending college. (Sunday, December 28)

This evening my whole family including Ronnie sat around and watched TV. Since Ronnie is without a girlfriend and has been home these past few nights. (December 30)

I am getting some orange juice in a few minutes to celebrate the New Year. (December 31)

This afternoon I watched the very exciting Cotton Bowl game between TCU and Air Force

Academy. The battle ended in a scoreless tie. (Thursday, January 1, 1959)

This afternoon I just sat around reading the book The Memoirs of Harry S. Truman. (January 2)

Today Ronnie made his departure to school after a two-week vacation. In a way I sort of hate to see him go because I will miss his meal. (January 3) [Mother prepared more of their favorite meals while Ron was home.]

I spent the afternoon studying my bookkeeping to try to have some papers ready to be checked when I go back to college tomorrow. (Sunday, January 4)

I have been entertaining myself with an evening of listening to sports on my radio. It included a Coyote basketball game, a boxing match, and sports news. (January 7)

I stayed out at the store this evening so I could listen to my daddy converse with longtime customers Mr. and Mrs. R. A. David. (January 10)

Tonight I listened to a Coyote basketball game against Arlington. The Coyotes won in a close game. (January 13)

This evening I went over to the Parker Square Theater to see "The High and Mighty." It was the most dramatic, suspenseful movie I've seen in quite a spell. (January 17)

At this time sleet mixed with snow is falling rapidly. (January 20)

Due to icy road conditions, I could not go to prayer meeting tonight. I certainly hated to miss it. (Wednesday, January 21)

The weather today was a little better than the blizzard conditions yesterday. The temperatures were in the 30s instead of the 20s. (January 22)

This evening I had a surprise visit from Mrs. Lucas and Dave Devers. The latter had arrived from Clovis, New Mexico where he is stationed in the Air Force. (January 23) [Dave Devers probably met Mrs. Lucas while stationed at SAFB.]

I spent the entire afternoon studying and working on income tax problems. (January 24)

Ronnie came home (from Texas A&M) late tonight. I was informed that he is going to Midwestern University next semester. (January 25)

Rod went back to Texas A&M to complete his senior year. Ron enrolled at Midwestern University for three classes and worked full-time at the Texas Highway Department surveying and drafting. He drove a state pickup to and from work.

I have just completed my studies in the "Income Tax Procedure" chapter. (Wednesday, February 4)

Tonight I took about 30 minutes of my time from my studies to watch "The Red Skelton Show." It was really entertaining. (February 5)

This morning I had a severe pain in my hip. I thought then for sure I would have to see a doctor. (February 6)

Tonight I attended the 15th Annual Court of Honor of Scout Troop 6 at Grant Street Methodist Church. I was "dishonorably" awarded Assistant Scout Master Code Certification. (Monday, February 9)

This evening I discovered that I had been guilty of forgetting that today was my mother's birthday. She is now 45 years old. (February 11)

Tonight I had my favorite dessert, ice cream and apple pie. (February 12) [His three favorite desserts seemed to depend on which one he had eaten most recently.]

Tonight I heard a very thrilling bi-district championship basketball game between the Coyotes and Grand Prairie. Trailing most of the game by 8 to 10 points, the Pack pulled it out of the fire to win 48-45. (February 13)

This afternoon I spent all my time working on some of the supplemental problems in the income tax book. (Sunday, February 15)

Since there was no prayer meeting at the church due to the annual study course held at First Baptist Church, I listened to a religious program on my radio. (February 18)

Tonight I went to visit the Troop 6 weekly meeting. I made arrangements with a couple of boys to come to my house Saturday afternoon for their Morse code test. (February 19)

This afternoon I worked with two boys on their Morse code test. Only one of them passed. (Saturday, February 21)

This evening I listened to one of my favorite programs "Party Line." They had a very interesting discussion on mental illness. (February 24)

This evening my mother fixed me one of my favorite desserts, blackberry pie. Man, it was delicious. (February 26)

Today I reached another milestone, I graduated from Draughon's Business College. It was the biggest thrill of my life! I was told that my diploma would be ready to be picked up on Monday. (Friday, February 27, 1959)

AN INCREDIBLE BOY AND A REMARKABLE MAN

This afternoon I worked with a boy on his Morse code test. He had failed the test last week. He failed again. (February 29)

This afternoon Ronnie and I threw passes and kicked his football. I certainly could tell that I was out of shape. (Sunday, March 1)

As I write this I am resting after a long hard day of babysitting. Thank goodness this is the last day to babysit until Saturday. (March 2)

I spent the afternoon reading last month's issue of "Sport" magazine. I really enjoyed it. (Sunday, March 7)

This evening a remarkable and inspiring incident occurred in our church. There was a Spiritual Awakening. This is the second time this has happened this year. (Sunday, March 8)

This evening I attended the first of four nights of a study course at our church. The adults and young people are studying the same book titled Personal Soul Winning. (March 9)

I got out of the house for a change. I went over to the Olympic and hanged out for about an hour and ten minutes. (March 10)

This afternoon I went over to the shoe shop on Grant St. to have one of my shoes repaired. It was partly torn and thus had to be sewed up. (March 11) [Kenneth Edmonds was the shoe repairman and was a friend of Daddy and Ron.]

Tonight I watched Part I of a play based on Ernest Hemingway's best-selling novel For Whom The Bell Tolls on TV. (March 12)

I've just watched a dramatic war movie "30 Seconds Over Tokyo." (March 14)

This evening I along with the rest of my family watched one of our favorite programs on

TV, "The Red Skelton Show." (Monday, March 17)

Tonight I practiced with my church piano accompanist, Wanda Battenfield, on a couple of hymns we are to play during the Prelude of the Sunday morning service. (March 18)

After lunch I went over to the church to practice on my marimba the music for Sunday. (March 19)

Tonight I took my bath and shaved to be ready to go to Fort Worth with Butch in the morning. (March 20)

I had a wonderful time with Sonny at his workshop. Along with Uncle John and Cousin Ivan who both work for Sonny, I kidded around with all of them. (March 21)

This morning the observance of Youth Week began with the Intermediate and Youth Departments in charge of the morning worship service. I played a couple of songs on my marimba. (Sunday, March 22)

This evening I went to the Intermediate and Young People skating party at Sand Beach. I certainly had a wonderful time. (March 23)

This evening at prayer meeting I was asked to play again next Sunday night at church. Having agreed to play, I made arrangements with my accompanist, Pearl Conner, to practice next Sunday afternoon. (March 25)

I stayed out here at the house for two hours practicing on the songs I will play Sunday night. (March 27)

I had a terrible experience this evening. After practicing for over two hours, I discovered that it came to no avail as I made numerous mistakes while playing in the worship service tonight. (Sunday, March 29) [Shelby usually played well.]

I just sat around tonight and read the current issue of "Newsweek" magazine. (March 30)

This evening for supper we had fish sticks, blackeye peas, cornbread, and fried potatoes. Um-m-m-m. (Friday, April 3)

Tonight I went over to Parker Square Theater to see "Friendly Persuasion." It was really a fine movie. (April 4)

This afternoon I passed the time away reading "Sport's Baseball Preview" and listening to my radio. (April 5)

I am sitting here on my bed wondering how I will meet my 23rd birthday emotionally tomorrow. (April 7)

Well today was my 23rd birthday. It did not bother me after reading an article in the newspaper emphasizing a man my age is still a spry youngster. (Wednesday, April 8)

I am sitting here at my desk "digging" the sounds of the U. S. Navy Band on my radio. It is real gone! (April 9)

Tonight I watched a tense, dramatic play on "Playhouse 90." The title was "The Day Before Atlanta." (April 10)

Today I watched the first televised major league baseball game of the year. The Milwaukee Braves beat the Pittsburgh Pirates 4-3. (Saturday, April 11)

This afternoon Mother and I worked about two hours putting up stock in the store. (April 15)

Today Mother had to babysit Steve because Aunt Ruth, who usually cares for Steve, was ill. (April 16)

This evening I went over to the Olympic and purchased a "Newsweek" magazine and spent some time reading it. (April 17)

I started back to work at the store after a week's absence due to my taking care of Steve who was sick. (April 27)

This afternoon my dad got off three hours early because the employees and students at Midwestern State University celebrated the passing of a state bill to make the school a four-year state-supported university. (Thursday, April 30)

This evening I viewed a World Heavyweight Championship fight between Champion Floyd Patterson and challenger Brian London. Patterson won by a KO in the eleventh round. (May 1)

I am sitting here at my desk enjoying the sounds of rock and roll. Ronnie is reading a western novel titled The Relentless Gun. (May 3)

[Shelby's 1959 diary ends. He had diaries in later years, but Ron only has January 1 to February 4 of 1987, February 7 to December 31 of 1996, a few months of 2002, the last half of 2003, and a few months of 2004. Selected entries will be forthcoming in later chapters.]

On May 23, Rod graduated from Texas A&M with a bachelor of science in geological engineering, but he had to stay on campus a few days to finish the *1959 Aggieland Yearbook* as editor of the publication. He had already accepted a job as a geophysicist with Pan American Petroleum Corporation, which was the exploration and production arm of Standard Oil of Indiana. However, before Rod could report to Pan American in Houston, he had to complete six weeks of ROTC training at Fort Sill Artillery Base in Lawton Oklahoma.

In late May, Jim Stepp finished the tenth grade at WFSH and David finished the seventh grade.

AN INCREDIBLE BOY AND A REMARKABLE MAN

After completing his training at Fort Sill, Rod received his officer's commission to second lieutenant on July 31 and then drove to Houston and reported to Pan American on August 3. As a newly commissioned officer, Rod chose the option of serving only six months of active duty to begin in November and end in May of 1960. Pan Am was okay with him working from August to November and then taking six months leave for military service.

Rod was excited about having a good job with a good company and for the first time in his life having a steady source of income. He was looking forward to getting the six-month active tour of duty behind him so he could concentrate his efforts on learning the job of a geophysicist.

Shelby worked in the store and helped care for Steve. Ron completed his three courses at Midwestern State University (MSU).

Summer 1959, Ron bought a 1957 Chevrolet Bel Air sedan, which was the same color as the one his daddy had bought two years earlier. Ron went to summer school at MSU and completed two courses, worked full-time at the Texas Highway Department (THD), and played softball with Lloyd for Downtown Baptist. They played in the church state playoffs in Houston but lost in the semifinals. Rod came to one of the games that they won. Rod invited Ron and Lloyd to a party that night, and they met his future girlfriend Claudia Buckalew from Conroe, Texas.

Shortly after beginning work at Pan Am, Rod was informed that if he worked for one year before taking leave to complete his six-month military service, Pam Am would accrue his time for company benefits. Rod contacted the army personnel service at Fort Hood and requested his starting date for active duty be changed to August 1960. His request was approved, and he was told that new orders would be issued.

Ron went to a wedding with Mother and Ruby, and his ex-fiancée was there. She came over and visited before the ceremony started, and she seemed to be happy. Pat Wright, the bride of the wedding, had lived across the street from the L. R. Stepp family from 1947 to 1954. For some reason, Shelby did not go with them to the wedding. He usually had several options for his evening social activities. Pat was an ex-girlfriend of Rennie Havens.

In September, Ron took three courses and worked full-time at the THD and started dating his future wife, Jeane Curfman. Jim Stepp started eleventh grade at WFSH, and David began the eighth grade in Zundy.

Shelby's Los Angeles Dodgers won the National League and in October beat the Chicago White Sox in six games to win the World Series. Shelby went to the home games of the Coyote football team and listened to the away games on his radio. They played for the state championship, but they lost to Corpus Christi Ray, 6–20.

The seven Stepp boys got together on Christmas morning for the last time. Their relationships were continuing to change, but they remained much like brothers. In January, Ron was notified by the Wichita Falls draft board that he would soon be drafted for military service because he was not taking enough college course hours each semester to be exempted from the draft. Ron completed the three courses at MSU, continued working at the THD, awaited being drafted, and dated Jeane. Shelby continued to look for employment.

Ron talked to the US Army recruiting sergeant in Wichita Falls about his desire to go to Officer Candidate School (OCS) at Fort Sill. He was told that if he enlisted for three years before he was drafted, he could go to OCS after basic training and apply for six months active duty after graduating from OCS. That would result in his serving a total of thirteen or fourteen months active duty. He immediately signed up.

On February 16, 1960, Ron reported to the army entrance center in downtown Dallas. After completing a bank of tests, he was told that his test results qualified him for the Army Security Agency School in Fort Devens, Massachusetts. Ron declined. Three hours later, the recruiting sergeant from Wichita Falls arrived and tried to talk him into going to the ASA School. Again, Ron declined.

Early the next morning, Ron joined a group of recruits in boarding a train that took them to Fort Carson, Colorado, to begin basic combat training. While he was there, Rod married Claudia Buckalew on April 16, 1960. Of course, Ron could not get a pass to be in the wedding.

Back in Wichita Falls, Shelby was still looking for employment but having no luck. He did enjoy working in the store, but the store was soon to be closed.

AN INCREDIBLE BOY AND A REMARKABLE MAN

Ron completed basic combat training, which was conducted in ice and snow during the first four weeks. Those few who had applied for OCS were told that the first sergeant of their battery had been arrested and was being held in jail awaiting trial, and that neither he nor his replacement had processed the OCS applications. Ron was also told that he could apply for OCS at his next duty station.

After basic training, Ron was able to spend three days in Wichita Falls before reporting for advanced training at Fort Sill, Oklahoma. Mother and Jeane met him at the bus station. Shelby had to stay at the store. Later when Shelby gave Ron his special hug,[6] Ron sat down and told him about some of the army training he had done. Having seen many WWII movies, Shelby understood most of what Ron told him. Ron enjoyed visiting family and friends, especially Jeane, for three days and then reported to his training outfit, C Battery, Fifth Training Battalion at Fort Sill on May 9, 1960.

Ron's eight weeks of training in field artillery were repeats of what he had learned in ROTC at Texas A&M and ROTC Summer Camp at Fort Sill. Early on he was assigned to drive one of the two-and-a-half-ton trucks to carry troops and pull a 105 mm howitzer when they went to the firing range.

Ron was able to get a pass most weekends and go home for a day and a half. It was only sixty miles from Fort Sill to Wichita Falls. *When Ron requested an application for OCS, he was told that he would have to wait until he arrived at his permanent duty station.* After the fifth week of training, Ron was told that his next duty station would be in West Germany. That meant that he would be in Germany without Jeane for an unknown period but probably three or four months. His new total time of active duty would be about eighteen months, but that would still be better than two years. Ron never got to talk to the recruiting sergeant about all the negative aspects of what he had told Ron about applying for OCS compared to what Ron had experienced in his efforts to apply for OCS.

In late May, Jim Stepp finished eleventh grade at WFSH, and David finished the eighth grade in Zundy.

Jeane and Ron got engaged and then got married on June 25. Rod was best man. They had a two-day honeymoon at Lake Murray near

Ardmore, Oklahoma. On July 2, Ron was awarded the "Outstanding Soldier of the Fifth Training Battalion" and "Honor Graduate" of C Battery. On July 3, Ron said goodbye to Jeane, Mother, and Steve and boarded a train in Lawton for Fort Dix, New Jersey, via Chicago and Philadelphia. Two days later, he boarded the USNS Darby near Fort Dix on July 5 and arrived at Bremerhaven, West Germany, nine days later. He then went by train to join his army outfit.

Cousin Jerry Ewing and his wife, Claudia, moved to Dallas, and Shelby would only see him a few more times on holidays and Ewing reunions. Jerry and Shelby always enjoyed each other when they got together. Another close relationship was now long distant.

Rod received orders for his army tour of duty, but it was different from what he had been told it would be. Instead of serving six months starting in August 1960, it was for starting a two-year tour of duty beginning April 25, 1961, at Fort Bliss, El Paso, Texas. The Berlin Crisis was changing tours of duty for hundreds of thousands of current and near future US military personnel including Rod and Ron.

Ron's outfit, A battery Third Howitzer Battalion, Thirty-Fifth Field Artillery, Seventh Army, was in Grafenwöehr for their annual one-month firing range training, which ended with a standard battery firing test. Their weapons were M55 self-propelled eight-inch howitzers mounted on tracks. When they returned to their military base at Peden Barracks in Wertheim, West Germany, Ron was assigned to the Fire Direction Center as the computer. Wertheim was a "fairy tale" village with a castle on a hill overlooking downtown, narrow cobblestone streets, and tall stone towers. It was also on the Main River (second largest river in West Germany).

Ron went to First Sergeant Albright and asked about applying for OCS and was told that he would be required to go to the Noncommissioned Officers Academy in Bad Tölz for one month of training and testing before being eligible to apply for OCS. It was not known as to how long it would be before he might go to the NCO Academy. To be qualified to go there, he had to be at least private first class. He could not be promoted to PFC until October 16 at the earliest. Also, he could not be certain as to how long after he graduated from the NCO Academy it would be before he could go to OCS.

But the clincher was that Ron was informed that recently the army had changed the regulation setting the minimum term for active duty for an OCS graduate from six months to two years. Ron wrote Jeane and updated her on the OCS fiasco, asked her to get an airline ticket to fly to Frankfurt, West Germany, and told her that he would meet her there. They could live on the local economy in Wertheim until quarters became available on post at Peden Barracks. Also, he explained that they were stuck with serving the full three years of active duty and that they would not return to Fort Sill until mid-July 1962. Also, Ron told Jeane that he understood that her parents would be concerned that their eighteen-year-old daughter would be gone overseas for almost two years.

Jeane promptly replied by mail that her dad had purchased a plane ticket from Oklahoma City to Frankfurt with Sabena Airlines and that he and her mother would drive her to Oklahoma City. In late August, Ron rented a two-room apartment in downtown Wertheim because quarters were not available on post at that time. Ron arranged for his daddy to purchase his 1957 Chevrolet after Jeane left home because they could not afford to pay to have it shipped overseas. So, Daddy ended up getting the dream car he wanted at a price he could afford. And Ron continued to pay for the insurance on the Chevy.

Jeane arrived at Rhein-Main Airport in Frankfurt on September 2. Ron remembers watching the 1960 Olympics men's one-hundred-meter dash on a TV in a store window while standing on a sidewalk the day before. Jeane and Ron spent three nights in a downtown hotel (Hotel Frankfurter Hof), ate at several restaurants, and window-shopped. They went by rail to Wertheim and enjoyed the scenery all along the Main (pronounced "Mine") River. They began their twenty-nine-month life together in Wertheim.

Back in Wichita Falls, Shelby had an extraordinary first and last experience in his life. *He drove an automobile.* He got behind the wheel of his daddy's '57 Chevy Bel Air, which was parked on the HHBC parking lot a few feet from the Stepp driveway. David sat in the middle of the front seat and started the car and put the Powerglide automatic transmission in gear. Steve stood up in the seat to the right of David. Shelby steered the car onto York Street and turned left while David handled the accelerator and brake pedals. After a short distance, Shelby turned left onto Hayes Road and shortly turned left onto an alley at the back of the parking lot and turned left again onto the parking lot back to where the trip began.

Shelby enjoyed driving so much that he repeated that short drive three more times. Then on the fifth trip after turning left onto York Street, Shelby steered straight down York Street one long block and turned left onto Garfield Road. He then drove a short block and turned left onto Avenue Q and steered past Aunt Ruby's house. She happened to be out on her front porch and saw Shelby, David, and Steve motoring along with Shelby at the wheel.

After driving the long block on Avenue Q, Shelby turned left onto Hayes Road, and then after steering a short distance, he turned right onto the alley and then turned left onto the parking lot and back to the spot where the car was parked before. The total distance of the trip was about 0.8 miles.

Aunt Ruby drove up while they were sitting in the car talking and laughing about Shelby "driving" a car. She scolded Shelby and David about endangering their lives and that of Steve who would turn five in a few days. But Shelby thought the thrill of "driving" a car was worth whatever punishment he might receive.

In early September, Jim Stepp started his senior year at WFSH and David began the ninth grade in Zundy. Steve would be six on September 25, but he would not start first grade until next year. Shelby was still looking for work, missing going to school, doing his exercises, and reading the local newspaper daily, making weekly visits to family and friends, playing his marimba, going to movies, watching TV, listening to music on his radio and record player, and attending church.

The New York Yankees played the Pittsburgh Pirates in the 1960 World Series. The Pirates won game 7 on a walk-off homer by Bill Mazeroski. Despite losing the series, the Yankees scored fifty-five runs, the most runs scored by any one team in World Series history, and more than twice as many as the Pirates, who scored twenty-seven. The Yankees won three blowouts (16–3, 10–0, and 12–0), while the Pirates won four close games (6–4, 3–2, 5–2, and 10–9) to win the World Series.[7] Shelby and Rod had nothing to cheer about as their LA Dodgers finished fourth in the National League with a record of eighty-two wins and seventy-two losses.

Ron was promoted to private first class (E3) on October 16, 1960. His battery had been selected by USAREUR command to provide demonstrations of field artillery in battle conditions at the NATO demonstration in Wiesbaden in late October. His battery had been cleaning and painting all weapons, vehicles, and equipment for two weeks. They worked long hours each day and night. Ron did not have much casual time with Jeane for four weeks.

Jeane shopped on the post at Peden Barracks at the PX and commissary, and she bought bakery items and some meats at the bakery and butcher shops near their apartment. Their favorite meat was wienerschnitzel.

"A" battery drove a convoy of howitzers[8] and other battery vehicles eighty-five miles to Wiesbaden on October 24, and they conducted demonstrations on October 25 and 27. There were officers and high-ranking noncommissioned officers from all fourteen NATO countries[9] in attendance including many generals. As computer for the Fire Direction Center (FDC), Ron called out the numerous fire commands over the loudspeakers in his Texas drawl during the demonstrations. The English probably did not understand him any better than the Germans and French. "A" battery received a commendation for their demonstrations and returned to Peden Barracks. The night they arrived home, First Sergeant Albright informed Ron that in two weeks he was going to the USAREUR NCO Academy in Bad Tölz for four weeks.

Ron had a buddy in FDC named John Bozeman who lived with his wife, Eleanor, in the top level of a three-level home owned by a German widow named Frau Kathe Albert. The couple was from California. John told Ron that a US Army couple living on the second level were going back stateside soon. Ron and Jeane met with Frau Albert and signed up to move in when the rooms were vacated. The second level had a bedroom, living room with a door to a balcony, which overlooked the Main River, and a kitchen. The bathroom in the hall on the second level was for both military couples.

Ron graduated from USAREUR Noncommissioned Officers Academy on December 16, 1960, and ranked tenth in the class of 163. Much like in Fort Carson, Colorado, most of his training was in ice and snow at Bad Tölz. US Army Special Forces troops were also in training there. When Ron got back to Wertheim, he found that John, Eleanor, and Jeane had moved everything into their new home. It was the beginning of a wonderful experience with the Bozemans for ten months and Frau Albert for twenty-six months. Jeane soon learned that Frau Albert's husband had been killed in WWII.

Ron and Jeane celebrated their first Christmas in Germany with John, Eleanor, and Frau Albert.

Mother began to operate the store with some help from Shelby, but it would not be for an extended period. Uncle Louis was making plans for M&M Manufacturing that would preclude his working in Fort Worth. He planned to lease Daddy's building and open a M&M workshop there.

Ron graduated from the USAREUR Special Weapons School on January 13, 1961.

There he learned to assemble nuclear warheads in eight-inch artillery shells.

On February 11, 1961, a son was born to Rod and Claudia. They named him David Randall. Also, Shelby's mother celebrated her forty-seventh birthday on that date.

On February 19, Eddie Lee Ewing died in Wichita Falls at the age of seventy-seven. His funeral service was held at HHBC and was well attended. Ron was not able to come home for his grandpa's service.

The Stepps and Bozemans took a five-day winter trip to Berchtesgaden, West Germany. On the first day, they went to Bad Tölz to show Jeane and Eleanor where John and Ron attended the NCO Academy. They spent the first night in Vaduz, Liechtenstein. The second day, they drove through the scenic Alps to Innsbruck, Austria. While in Innsbruck, they watched bobsled competition. Afterward as Ron and Jeane walked holding hands down a nearby icy path, Jeane slipped and fell on her back pulling Ron down on top of her, and Ron rode her down the icy slope. Fortunately, they were both bundled up with four layers of clothing including thick overcoats. Ron said to Jeane, "Those spectators are probably saying, 'Look at those crazy Americans acting like they are bobsledding.'"

They drove on to Berchtesgaden and spent two nights at the US Army General Walker Hotel. They went skiing the second day and toured Hitler's Eagles Nest and Salzburg, Austria, the third day. In Salzburg, they toured the home of Wolfgang Amadeus Mozart. On the fourth day, they ate breakfast in a small cozy country cabin tucked away amid four mounds of ice and snow on the way to Linz, Austria. It was run by a mother and daughter. The mother reminded Ron of Al Capp's Mammy Yokum character. The meal was very excellent, the room and furnishings were cute and quaint, and the atmosphere was pleasant.

They spent the last night in Linz, Austria, and then drove back to Wertheim via Passau and Regensburg alongside the Danube River, Nurnberg, and Wurzburg.

In mid-March, Jeane was told that she was three months pregnant. Their baby would be due in September. Ron had picked out a name for his first son during his senior year at Texas A&M while in his dorm after seeing the movie *Shane* starring Alan Ladd. He wrote down "Ron Alan Stepp." Jeane liked the name. If they had a daughter, her name would be Dana Lea.

On April 8, 1961, Shelby celebrated his twenty-fifth birthday. Also, it was Rod's twenty-fourth.

* * * * *

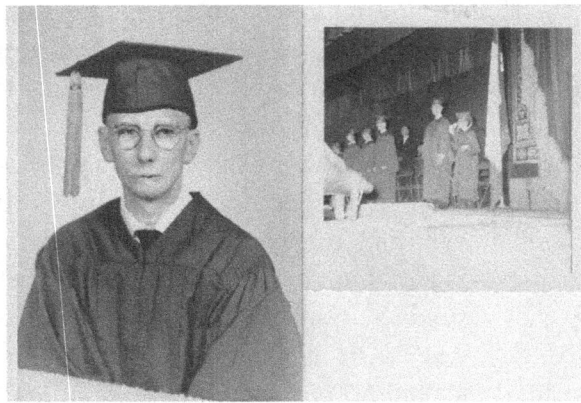

Shelby's graduation from WFSH in May 1956.
He is on the right on stage.

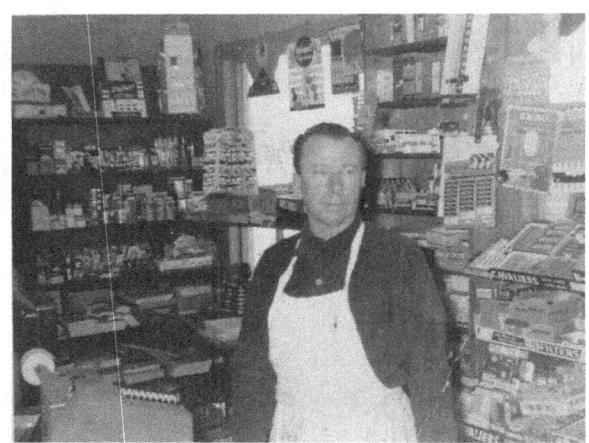

Lee Roy Stepp in his grocery store at 2604 Grant St. in 1956. Shelby stocked the shelves and swept the floors part-time from 1956 to 1961.

AN INCREDIBLE BOY AND A REMARKABLE MAN

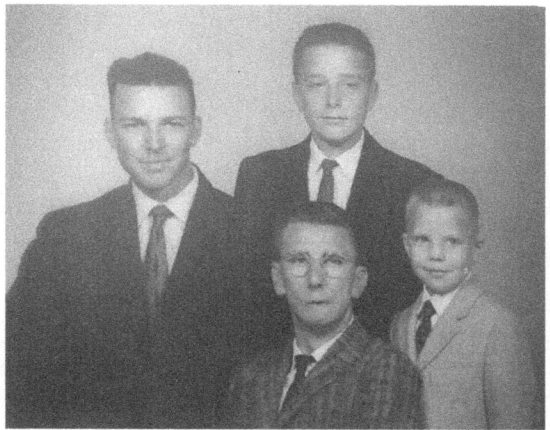

Ron, Shelby, David, and Steve on Ron's wedding day June 25, 1960

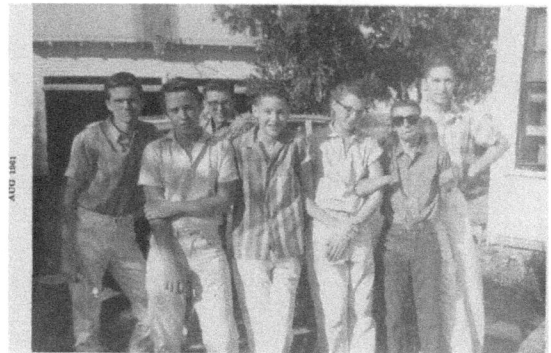

Uncle Ike and his newspaper boys including Shelby in August 1961

---

[1] 2803 York Street, Wichita Falls, Texas, November 17, 1957

Dear Ronald,

With my morale partially split by Oklahoma's shocking defeat by the Notre Dame Irish, I am still able to express with little delightfulness to see the Aggies sovereignty crumbled. I have been waiting for quite a while to retaliate against Aggie braggarts like you. Any dirty, lowdown, yellowbellied guys like you have found it a fact that Texas A&M does not have an invincible team. It wasn't luck that beat you. It was Rice's stout defense. Of course, you haven't seen anything yet until Texas University invades. Brother, they're going to clobber the daylights out of you. Having been shaken up by the Owls (Rice), the Aggies will still be so stunned that the Longhorns will kick them all over the field. As far as the Cotton Bowl is concerned my prediction is that either Texas or Rice will get the nod.

Oh yes! There is one small inquiry pertinent to sports. I had a Sporting News edition along with a coupon from a St. Louis firm under the chinaware on the buffet. It was there during your last home visit. One day while searching for something to read I thought of that newspaper. I went to get it but it was not there and neither was the coupon. This took place ironically a few days after your last visit. Did you by any chance take them back to school? Comrade, let me emphasize that my name and address was printed on the newspaper. If you have it by all means bring it home when you come back next week. Whichever property bears my name you should always ask for permission to utilize them for your convenience.

Well, gutless Aggie, that's about all I have to say until after the Texas Longhorns torture you on Thanksgiving Day. Until that time, Adios.

Your (Hate'em Aggies) brother,
Shelby R. Stepp [Ron had neither his magazine nor coupon.]

2   Gerald was a younger brother of one of Rod's and Ron's buddies Larry Phillips. He was going steady with Jeane Curfman at that time. Later he was ordained as a Baptist minister.
3   *Suspicion* was the title of an American television mystery drama series that aired on the NBC from 1957 through 1958.
4   A deadly F3 tornado with record wind gusts of 450 kph (281 mph) struck Wichita Falls, killing one and injuring fourteen.
5   Chart of accounts in balance sheet order. Bookkeepers and accountants use this report to consolidate all the T-accounts into one document and double-check that all transactions were recorded in proper journal entry format.
6   When Shelby hugged family adults and close friend adults, depending on their height, he placed his face on their chest, abdomen, or waist and wrapped his arms tightly around their sides above the waist or lower and squeezed for five to ten seconds.
7   The Series MVP was Bobby Richardson of the Yankees, the only time in history that the award has been given to a member of the losing team, though the rules were different at this time. Votes had to be in by the start of the eighth inning of game 7, at which point the Yankees were in the lead, and this was the first

AN INCREDIBLE BOY AND A REMARKABLE MAN

    time since the series MVP award was created in 1955 that the team leading at that point did not go on to win.

[8] The M55 self-propelled eight-inch Howitzer had two 190-gallon gasoline tanks and got 0.43 miles per gallon. Top speed was thirty miles per hour. The convoy to Wiesbaden would have averaged about twenty-five miles per hour and taken about three and a half hours. Each M55 Howitzer would have used about 200 gallons of fuel.

[9] Twelve countries took part in the founding of NATO in 1949: Belgium, Canada, Denmark, France, Iceland, Italy, Luxembourg, the Netherlands, Norway, Portugal, the United Kingdom, and the United States. In 1952, Greece and Turkey joined NATO.

CHAPTER 6

Middle Adult Years: Twenty-Five to Fifty (1961–1986)

In early 1961, the East German government sought a way to stop its population leaving for the West. The East German government began secretly stockpiling building materials for the erection of the Berlin Wall.

The West had advance intelligence about the construction of the wall. An intercept of SED[1] communications informed the West that there were plans to begin blocking all foot traffic between East and West Berlin. It was viewed as the first step in a plan to close the border, which turned out to be correct.

Ron was promoted to specialist four (E4) on April 17, 1961.

About this time, Rod and Claudia packed everything they owned, and with baby Randall, they drove to El Paso, and Rod reported for duty at Fort Bliss on April 26, 1961, to begin three months of officers basic training.

In late May, Jim Stepp graduated from WFSH and David finished the ninth grade in Zundy. Aunt Ruby divorced Uncle Sonny about this time and married J. D. Faulkenberry. They lived in Ruby's house on Avenue Q.

Ron and Jeane became friends of Master Sergeant Carl and Faye Cotton who were originally from Arkansas. They often visited, and when Ron and Carl were gone, which was often, Jeane and Faye spent much time together. Carl and Faye had two young sons, Carl Don and Barry.

The Berlin Crisis began to heat up after President Kennedy met with Soviet Premier Khrushchev at a summit meeting in Vienna, Austria, on June 3–4, 1961. Khrushchev reissued the Soviet ultimatum to sign a separate peace treaty with East Germany and thus end the existing four-power agreements guaranteeing American, British, and French rights to access West Berlin and the occupation of East Berlin by Soviet forces. However, this time, he did so by issuing a deadline of December 31, 1961. The three powers of the West responded that any unilateral treaty could not affect their responsibilities and rights in West Berlin.

Ron and Jeane with army buddy Andy Wilburn from Shelbyville, Texas, left Wertheim on July 11 on a two-week trip to Rome and back in their 1959 Volkswagen. They drove through southern West Germany, Switzerland, France, Spain, Monaco, Italy, and Austria. They camped out all except two nights. The first night, they camped out beside the Neckar River in Heidelberg, and Ron listened to the MLB All-Star Game.

The highlights of their trip were the majestic Alps, the French Riviera, Monaco (toured the palace of Princess Grace), the Italian Riviera, the Leaning Tower of Pisa, tours of Rome, Florence, Venice, and the bullfights in Barcelona. While standing in San Marco Square in Venice, Jeane recognized a high school classmate passing by in a gondola, but Ron could not get Jeane to holler at her.

Ron wrote that the Germans, Swiss, and Austrians were very friendly, the Spaniards were friendly, but the French were discourteous, and the Italians were ambivalent. On July 25, they drove through Munich which is 250 miles from Vienna where Kennedy and Khrushchev met seven weeks earlier. They arrived in Wertheim late that night. Shelby would never see much of the world outside of Texas.

On July 25, President Kennedy delivered a television speech in Washington in which he reiterated that the United States was not looking for a fight. He also announced that he would ask Congress for an additional $3.25 billion for military spending, mostly on conventional weapons. He wanted six new divisions for the Army and two for the Marines, and he announced plans to triple the draft and to call up the reserves. Kennedy proclaimed: "We seek peace, but we shall not surrender." Premier Khrushchev was reported to be angered by Kennedy's speech and said that Kennedy's military buildup threatened war.

On the same day of President Kennedy's speech, Rod completed his officers basic training at Fort Bliss, and five days later, he reported for duty at the 4th Missile Battalion, 562nd Artillery in Duncanville, Texas. This was headquarters for the Dallas-Fort Worth Defense Area, which had four Nike Hercules and Ajax Batteries under their command. These batteries were in Texas, at Denton, Terrell, Alvarado, and Mineral Wells. Their primary mission was to protect the Dallas-Fort Worth area against Russian bomber attacks. Each battery was equipped with about thirty missiles, both Ajax and Hercules. The Hercules had nuclear warheads that were larger than the bombs dropped on Hiroshima and Nagasaki. Each battery was manned with about 125 enlisted men, four warrant officers, and four commissioned officers.

With the Berlin Crisis intensifying, USAREUR issued orders for an adult from each US Army family stationed in Europe to drive or be driven the designated evacuation routes in preparation for quick departure when situations required. Ron and Jeane drove the evacuation route that Jeane would use in the event she received orders to evacuate.

Back in Wichita Falls, Shelby tried selling electric light bulbs in mid-1961, but he gave it up after five months of little income and difficulty communicating with customers. He read the newspaper daily and often listened to the news on his transistor radio, and he knew what the Berlin Crisis was. He also heard Jim and David talk about the air raid drills at school.

Uncle Louis leased Daddy's store space and opened a M&M Manufacturing Branch. Shelby inquired about working for him, but all the work required handling heavy steel sheet metal or operating heavy machinery or selling to customers. Shelby could do none of those jobs, so he continued to look for employment.

AN INCREDIBLE BOY AND A REMARKABLE MAN

On Saturday August 12, 1961, the leaders of East Germany met in a wooded area to the north of East Berlin, and Walter Ulbricht signed the order to close the border and erect a wall.

At midnight, the army, police, and units of the East German army began to close the border, and by morning on August 13, 1961, the border to West Berlin had been closed.

On August 30, 1961, in response to moves by the Soviet Union to cut off access to Berlin, President Kennedy ordered 148,000 guardsmen and reservists to active duty. In October and November, more Air National Guard units were mobilized, and 216 aircraft from the tactical fighter units flew to Europe in operation "Stair Step," the largest jet deployment in the history of the Air Guard.

In early September, Jim began his freshman year in the Corps of Cadets at Texas A&M, David started the tenth grade in WFSH, and Steve began the first grade at Sam Houston grade school.

In the middle of the night of September 9–10, Ron rushed Jeane to the Peden Barracks Dispensary. The medic on duty examined her and called Dr. Romano who chose not to come and examine her. He told the medic to take her to the US Army Hospital in Würzburg, which was about thirty miles from Peden Barracks. Ron followed the three-fourth-ton army ambulance in his Volkswagen. After about fifteen miles, the ambulance pulled off the highway and stopped. Ron got in the ambulance cab and watched the delivery through the back window of the cab. Soon they drove on to their destination. While in the hospital waiting room, a nurse came and told Ron that his son had died and that Jeane was all right physically. When Ron was allowed to see Jeane, they talked about many things, including the need to depend on God to see them through this heartrending loss, whether God would bless them with another child, where to bury their son, whether to save the name Ron Alan for their next son, etc. They decided to name their son Jon Michael, to have his body sent to Wichita Falls for burial by their parents, to lean on God, to publicly handle this loss in Christian manner that would be a testimony to their faith in Jesus Christ. The latter influenced them in dismissing any pursuit of bringing charges against Dr. Romano. They had given no thought about charging Dr. Romano for malpractice even though

Jeane did not like the way he treated her during the pregnancy, but they were asked by the hospital administrator about doing so. Ron called his parents and told them the pertinent information and asked them to call Jeane's parents.

The following day, which was a Monday, Ron was given time off duty to drive to Frankfurt and purchase a small casket at the US Army Post Exchange. He then made the arrangements for the body to be shipped to his folks. Ron brought Jeane home on Wednesday, September 14. Frau Albert gave Jeane loving care for several weeks. Jeane was soon back to her regular schedule including teaching four-year-olds in Sunday school at the Peden Barracks Chapel. She usually had about thirty-five pupils. Jon Michael was buried in Jeane's parents plot at Crestview Memorial Park. (All subsequent interments will be at Crestview Memorial Park unless otherwise stated.)

Ron was promoted to specialist five (E5) on October 18, 1961. That rank was equivalent to sergeant. His battery commander, Captain Mitchell, approached him about being recommended for an oral exam by an army promotion board for the purpose of qualifying for a promotion to second lieutenant. When Ron learned that he would have to sign up for another three-year tour of duty, he declined the recommendation.

Ron's battalion stayed combat ready and had combat readiness tests every two months. He joined a small group in making a reconnaissance of the Central Uplands of West Germany northeast of Frankfurt am Main defended by the US Army and West German troops. It was generally assumed by the commanders of these troops that the Fulda Gap was the most likely area that the Soviet army would attack first in the Central Uplands.

The four powers governing Berlin (Soviet Union, United States, United Kingdom, and France) had agreed at the 1945 Potsdam Conference that Allied personnel could move freely in any sector of Berlin. But on October 22, 1961, just two months after the construction of the wall, the US Chief of Mission in West Berlin, E. Allan Lightner, was stopped in his car (which had occupation forces license plates) while crossing at Checkpoint Charlie to go to a theater in East Berlin. The former army general Lucius D. Clay, US

President John F. Kennedy's special advisor in West Berlin, decided to demonstrate American resolve.

Clay sent an American diplomat, Albert Hemsing, to probe the border. While probing in a vehicle clearly identified as belonging to a member of the US Mission in Berlin, Hemsing was stopped by East German police asking to see his passport. Once his identity became clear, US Military Police were rushed in. The military police escorted the diplomatic car as it drove into East Berlin, and the shocked GDR[2] police got out of the way. The car continued, and the soldiers returned to West Berlin.

"Fallout Protection: What to Know and Do About Nuclear Attack" was an official US federal government pamphlet released in December 1961 by the US Department of Defense and the Office of Civil Defense ordered by President John F. Kennedy to "give the American people the facts they need to know about the dangers of a thermonuclear attack and what they can do to protect themselves."

Steve Stepp shared this memory from late 1961: "At the age of seven, I was snooping through the closet in David and Shelby's bedroom, and I came across a '78 LP record that contained an interview with Shelby. I got to thinking that he was somewhat of a celebrity. I also found an old *Jet* magazine[3] that had Shelby's picture on the cover. That just reinforced my belief that Shelby was a very special human being. He played his marimba on a telethon that Ken Curtis, who was cast as Festus Haggen in the TV show *Gunsmoke*, was hosting at one of the television stations in Wichita Falls. Shelby played two or three songs and ended in a flourish with the Marine fight song and raised both arms with enthusiasm at the finish. The overwhelming look on Ken Curtis's face was enough to bring tears to my eyes. I was so proud of my brother and still am to this day."

On Friday, March 9, 1962, David and his best friend, Larry White, and six other boys drove up to Mount Scott near Lawton, Oklahoma, in two cars. School was out that day because of Teachers Training Day at WFSH. After viewing the surrounding area from the top of Mount Scott, they started down the mountain on the winding paved roadway. Suddenly, the brakes on the car that David was in quit working. As the driver tried to slow the uncontrolled increasing speed of the car by scraping the right side of the car against the stone wall, he lost control of the car. Larry fell out of the car, and it rolled over on him. For the rest of his life, Larry was paralyzed from the waist down. David and others only had mild injuries. Larry was often visited by David and others in the following years.

Master Sergeant Carl Cotton was promoted to first sergeant of "A" Battery. Ron completed a chemical, biological, and radiological monitoring and survey course on April 27, 1962.

Shelby sold newspapers at Sheppard Air Force Base in 1962. Uncle Ike was a distributor for the *Wichita Daily Times* and *Record News*. He had several boys working for him delivering newspapers to residences. He took Shelby to SAFB each morning. At SAFB, Shelby often watched the B-52 Stratofortress bombers take off and land.

Ron was informed in early June that his tour of duty in West Germany was extended from July 5, 1962, to January 25, 1963, because of the Cuban Crisis. Rod was promoted to first lieutenant on July 31, 1962.

In September 1962, Jim began his sophomore year at Texas A&M, David was in the eleventh grade at WFSH, and Steve was in the second grade. In Denton, Rod was made commanding officer of his battery. In Wertheim, Ron was transferred to Headquarters Battery, Third Howitzer Battalion of the Thirty-Fifth Artillery, and was put in charge of the Battalion Fire Direction Center under Captain Sanders.

The *Stars and Stripes* American military newspaper became much more widely read during these times.

During the United States elections, the White House denied charges that it was ignoring dangerous Soviet missiles in Cuba just ninety miles away from Florida. But on October 14, an American U-2 surveillance plane on reconnaissance flights over Cuba took photographs that, over the next few days, were analyzed and showed that the Soviet Union was installing medium-range nuclear weapons in Cuba, capable of striking major US cities and killing tens of millions of Americans within minutes. With the photographs, the United States caught the Soviet Union building offensive nuclear missile bases in its backyard, and the two superpowers were now joined in the first direct nuclear confrontation in history.

In a televised address on October 22, 1962, President Kennedy informed the American people of the presence of missile sites in Cuba. When the United States put a naval blockade in place around Cuba, tensions mounted, and the world wondered if there could be a peaceful resolution to the crisis. Kennedy's speech drew wide support in Latin America and among United States' allies. The Pentagon continued plans for possible air strikes and a land invasion. Several Soviet vessels turned back from the quarantine line set by the naval blockade, and during a televised confrontation with the Soviet Union in the United Nations, the United States presented photographic proof of the missiles.

Ron's artillery battalion was deployed east of Schweinfurt for one of their semiannual two-week combat readiness exercises. They were getting frequent updates on the status of what was called "The October Crisis" or "The Cuban Crisis" and remained in combat readiness at all times. One night while in his sleeping bag, Ron was awakened by the loud sounds of tanks, trucks, and other vehicles moving into battle positions on either side of his battalion. It became more likely that they would soon be at war with Russia. After midnight on October 28, Ron was on duty in the battalion headquarters command post tent when a brigadier general came in and said Khrushchev had backed down and the crisis was over for now. Ron quickly initiated the spread of the good news.

In Denton, during this time, Rod's battery had received orders to make their missiles ready to fire and keep them ready. They created a perimeter of defense around their radar area and launch area, which were about a mile apart. All personnel were required to receive numerous immunizations. They were placed on *alert* status. No one could leave the post for several weeks until either Kennedy or Khrushchev backed down.

Shelby worried about the possibility of nuclear war as did most Americans. For some reason, those on active military duty were not as concerned as the American civilians about the possibility of a nuclear war.

On Sunday, October 28, the Soviets agreed to remove the missiles from Cuba. Negotiations for final settlement of the crisis continued for several days, but the immediate threat of nuclear war had been averted. On November 20, Kennedy announced, "I have today been informed by Chairman Khrushchev that all of the IL-28 bombers in Cuba will be withdrawn in thirty days… I have this afternoon instructed the Secretary of Defense to lift our naval quarantine." In addition, the United States agreed that it would never participate in an invasion of Cuba.

Because the US withdrawal of the Jupiter missiles from NATO bases in Italy and Turkey was not made public at the time, Khrushchev appeared to have lost the conflict and become weakened. The perception was that Kennedy had won the contest between the superpowers and that Khrushchev had been humiliated. That was as President Kennedy intended.

Ron was promoted to staff sergeant (E6) on November 13, 1962. Soon after, Ron and Jeane ordered a new 1963 Volkswagen Beetle with a sunroof. Since they had thought until June that they would be able to spend Christmas 1962 with family in Wichita Falls, they decided not to decorate their apartment for Christmas. They were not in the mood to celebrate Christmas. However, on Christmas Eve, a flatbed truck parked in front of their apartment. A Christmas tree was on the bed of the truck. The tree was brought up to their apartment. Frau Albert had ordered it. Jeane and Ron expressed to her their gratitude, and they immediately began to decorate the tree, and the next day, they celebrated the birth of Jesus. Frau Albert also brought them a German fruitcake[4] like she had baked for them on two other occasions. Frau Albert often gave them treats and did favors for them.

While Rod was stationed at the Nike missile site and after the Cuban Missile Crisis, Uncle Louis Watkins approached Rod about maybe joining him and Sonny at M&M. Louis was getting tired of driving back and forth from Wichita Falls to Fort Worth, but he realized that a solution might be to add a partner or manager in the Fort Worth plant. Louis offered to sell Rod 10 percent of the company (part of his 50 percent) if Rod would move to Fort Worth and become a partner in the business. Sonny agreed to give Rod 10 percent of his 50 percent, so the three-partner ownership would be 40-40-20. Sonny recognized that the company had potential, and he would be pleased to have Rod come to Forth Worth. However, Sonny was also worried about Rod leaving a good job with Pan American and about what would happen if the move did not work out for Rod. Sonny wanted to share the future if it worked out but also was anxious about the prospect of "what if it did not work out well." Louis recognized Rod's abilities and thought that Rod's presence would solve his "back and forth" problem, while also making the company even stronger.

Rod had enjoyed his two years with Pan American, and he looked forward to returning there after the army, but there was something gnawing at him about owning his own business. He had always felt that someday he would be "running my own business," and M&M might provide an entry into that vision.

The Lee Roy Stepp family moved from 2803 York Street to 3111 Avenue Q, which was a move of three city blocks. The house only had two bedrooms, but Daddy later added two bedrooms and a utility room. He did the carpenter work and painting himself. Shelby then had his own bedroom.

In early January, in blizzard conditions, Ron and Jeane drove their Volkswagen to Bremen, West Germany, and arranged for shipment from Bremerhaven to Newark Port in New Jersey, USA. On January 25, Ron and Jeane said goodbye to many friends including Frau Albert. Then army buddy Joe Catalano and his wife Gloria drove them 45 miles to Frankfurt where Ron and Jeane boarded a train and rode 240 miles to Bremerhaven. The next morning, they boarded the USNS Darby in blizzard conditions. The North Sea was covered with ice and snow the first twenty minutes of the trip. Two icebreaker ships cleared a path for their passage to the open waters of the North Sea.

Jeane was seasick the entire nine days of the trip. Ron went out on deck every day, but for only ten minutes each time because of the blizzard conditions. The meals were first class, but Jeane was not ever able to go to the dining room. Four days into the nine-day cruise, the captain of the ship said if Jeane's condition worsened, he would have to turn the ship back to the British Isles. Her condition did not improve, but it did not get worse. It was nine full days of misery for Jeane.

On February 4, Ron and Jeane saw the Statue of Liberty, and there was ice twenty feet out from the shore. They were taken to Fort Hamilton by bus and ate supper in the cafeteria. They selected roast beef with gravy, mashed potatoes with gravy, and whole kernel corn. When Ron finished his meal, he went back through the line and got the same meal again.

The next morning, Ron was processed out of the army. He smoked what he said would be his last cigarette ever.[5] Then they rode the subway to a shipping office in downtown New York City to get the papers needed to pick up their car in New Jersey. They took a taxi to Newark Port and picked up their Volkswagen. They had planned to have a brief visit with Joe Catalano's parents in Long Island, but they had already had enough of New York City. It seemed to them like a foreign country. They headed to Washington, DC, and spent the night in a Howard Johnson in College Park, Maryland, about ten miles from the Capitol in DC. They had an increasing desire to get back home with their families in Wichita Falls.

The following morning, they drove to the Capitol and took some photos of the White House, Capitol, Lincoln Memorial, Washington Monument, etc. They had intended to tour the Capitol, but home was calling louder, and they drove about fifteen miles to Alexandria, Virginia, to a restaurant for breakfast. The Southern waitresses in cowgirl skirts, vests, and hats made Ron feel at home. They dined on eggs, ham, grits, biscuits, gravy, and orange juice. It was a "yahoo" meal.

Jeane wanted to go to the Marine Corps Air Station in Havelock, North Carolina, for a quick visit with Barbara King Foster McGuire who was a bridesmaid in their wedding. They drove 350 miles to get there that evening and visited for about two hours. The next day, they drove 500 miles to a motel near Stone Mountain ten miles east of Atlanta, Georgia. The following morning, they had another good Southern breakfast, and then they drove 550 miles through Alabama and Mississippi to El Dorado, Arkansas, and spent the night in a motel. The next day, they would be *home*. They were more excited than ever as they talked about getting to visit their families the next day.

On February 9, Ron and Jeane drove 368 miles through southern Arkansas and North Texas. They arrived at Jeane's parents shortly after noon. Webb Curfman answered the doorbell with a mouthful of cheese and crackers, which prevented him from speaking as he hugged Jeane. After visiting several hours with Webb and Teddie Curfman, Ron and Jeane drove one mile to the L. R. Stepp home at 3111 Avenue Q and visited for several hours with Ron's parents, Shelby, David, and Steve. What a great time was had by all. Their futures were all very bright.

On April 8, Shelby got his first adult tricycle for his twenty-seventh birthday. It was more efficient and safer than his bicycle with training wheels. He rode it to homes of family and friends, movie theaters, the YMCA, Coyote football and basketball games, MSU basketball games, and the barbershop. Also, he occasionally went to the Wichita Falls Symphony Orchestra (WFSO) at the Memorial Auditorium. He had a lock and chain for security, a wire basket to carry items (transistor radio, newspaper, etc.), and a canvas bag to carry the items with him when he left his adult tricycle (trike). He wore a chain necklace, which held his keys. He rode his trike somewhere nearly every day. He often rode at night, which required a flashlight mounted on his handlebars. When he sat on a park bench at night to read a newspaper, he positioned his trike to enable using the flashlight as a reading light. Whatever the situation, Shelby always found a way to make do with what he had. Over the course of many years, friends and family often talked about seeing Shelby on his trike or sitting and reading his newspaper three or four miles from his home. All his trike trips were less than five miles.

Ron had contacted the Texas Highway Department (THD) by mail about employment when he got back home in Wichita Falls. In the return mail, he was told that he would be hired as a draftsman when he returned. Ron had planned to begin work at THD about two weeks after he and Jeane got back home, which would give him time to visit with the many family and friends in Wichita Falls and to drive to Denton and visit Rod and drive to Fort Worth to visit Sonny and Butch.

But when he arrived in Wichita Falls, THD called him to work two days later. THD had to meet a deadline for drafting plan work for multiple expressways in the Wichita Falls area for bidding contracts to be let in late February.

Rod was discharged from the army on April 25. He and Claudia had been looking forward to that day so they could go back to Houston and Pan Am. But while in Denton, they had often enjoyed visiting Sonny, and Sonny had enjoyed spending time with his first grandson. And the recent offer by his daddy and Uncle Louis to join them as partners at M&M weighed heavy on his mind. Rod finally decided it would be best for Claudia, who was almost three months pregnant, to return to Pan Am.

Ron got home from work one day, and Jeane told him that she had been in a car accident. She said that a car full of high school girls had run into the back of the Volkswagen while she was stopped at a traffic light on Kell Boulevard. Ron heard about a man named Jerry Allen who did good bodywork on vehicles. Ron drove the car out to Jerry's house north of Wichita Gardens, and Jerry repaired the rear bumper and decklid and spot painted the decklid. He did a good job at a good price. This was the beginning of a long friendship.

In early June, Ron began taking night courses at MSU while working full-time at THD. He played softball for the Downtown Baptist Church team, and they ended the season as church league champions. In August, they played in the Texas Church Playoffs in El Paso, but they lost in the semifinals.

Ron planned to finish his college work at Texas A&M while working full-time as a draftsman at THD in Bryan, Texas. However, before the summer was over, three THD engineers that Ron worked with convinced him to continue working at THD in Wichita Falls and finish his college work at MSU. All three engineers were graduates of Texas A&M. Jeane, her parents, Ron's parents, and Shelby strongly supported this option, so Ron relented. It worked out favorably for all concerned. Actually, the deciding factor in this important decision took place on July 3 when Jeane gave birth to her second son. He was given the name Ron Alan. Shelby became an uncle along with David and Steve.

The threesome of Shelby, Rod, and Ron did not reunite for an extended period. Rod and Ron were super busy for many months while Shelby's search for meaningful occupation continued.

After several months at Pan Am, Rod realized that he had to give the M&M option a try. If he was going to go broke in his own business, it would be better to do it while he was young. Times were good in the "oil patch," and Pan Am offered to give him a two-year leave of absence.

So, on August 3, Rod started to work at M&M Manufacturing. He became the sixth M&M employee in Fort Worth, along with Sonny, Jack Brown, Charlie York, Paul Henson, and cousin Ivan Stepp. Uncle Louis and Aunt Lydia Watkins and Cousin Paul Bond were the three employees in the M&M workshop in Wichita Falls. Rod began to make some of the basic sheet metal products and to get familiar with the plant operations and catalog of products. But he soon decided to designate every Thursday as "customer calling day." Rod's commitment to his "Customer Calling Thursdays" was his greatest contribution to the annual growth of sales at M&M his first two years. He also was the bookkeeper for the Fort Worth plant.

In September 1963, Jim began his junior year at Texas A&M, David was in the twelfth grade, and Steve was in the third grade. Ron took two courses at MSU and scheduled his forty hours of THD work around his course hours. Shelby made his nightly visits to the homes of family and friends, and he played his marimba often at HHBC, other churches, and other venues.

On November 5, 1963, Claudia gave birth to a daughter in Fort Worth, Texas, and she was named Rhonda Ann. On November 22, President Kennedy was assassinated in Dallas, Texas. On the same day, C. S. Lewis died in Oxford, England. He would later become one of Ron's two favorite authors of books on Christianity. The other author was Dietrich Bonhoeffer.

The Lee Roy Stepp family enjoyed Christmas 1963 together at Daddy's home. Mother cooked her usual "hen and dressing" dinner[6] with many sides and several pies. Gifts were opened, and favorite memories of past Christmases were shared. They all then went to the Curfman's home and opened more gifts there. No one enjoyed this Christmas day and night more than Shelby because he had missed Ron and Jeane the previous three Christmases, and for the first time, he got to enjoy Christmas with the Curfmans.

In 1964, Jerry and Rita Allen moved into a house across the street from the Lee Roy Stepp's house in the 3100 block of Avenue Q. Shelby started visiting them regularly, and they became two of Shelby's best friends for the rest of his life. They had two daughters, Cheryl and Christy, ages six and two. In October of 1965, they were blessed with a son whom they named Monte.

Shelby began working at the Opportunity Workshop for handicapped workers located on Armory Road near Midwestern Parkway in 1964. God had heard his prayers for a real job. That year, the following article appeared in Glenn Shelton's column of the *Wichita Falls Times*:

> He was a skinny bundle of energy. He had neither hands nor feet, but he worked tirelessly, sweeping floors, cleaning tools. "I have to force him to quit when the day is done," said Glen Fox, workshop supervisor. The man in question was born handi-capped, almost to the extent of the fabulous Helen Keller. A bizarre caricature of a human being, he nevertheless was happy in his work. And he worked like a machine, tirelessly, alone. "It is strange," said Fox, "but the half-hundred here in Opportunity Workshop, though physically handicapped, are on the whole happier than the so-called sound people. They are with their own. They like being together and working together."

In late May, David graduated from WFSH, Jim finished his junior year at A&M, and Steve finished third grade. Butch started working full-time at M&M in Fort Worth. He had always been interested in making mechanical and electrical things and in working with electronics. Over the years at M&M, he made valuable contributions to the growth and success of the company in the production area in charge of acquiring the machines and computers necessary to remain highly competitive.

In the summer of 1964, Ron took two courses at MSU while working full-time at THD. He played softball for Downtown Baptist Church, and at season end, they were church league champions. Ron still missed Shelby being batboy for his team.

In September 1964, Jim began his senior year at Texas A&M, and Steve was in the fourth grade. Ron took three courses at MSU and scheduled his forty hours of THD work around his course hours. He also became friends with Roger Bacon while working and going to school together. Roger's family had moved from Callisburg, Texas, to Wichita Falls in 1941, and the first people they met were Lee Roy and Sonny Stepp at Stepp Brothers Grocery-Service Station-Café. Roger remembers going inside the store and seeing a small boy with no hands or feet sitting on the countertop by the cash register.

Just before Christmas, Ron and Jeane drove on icy highways to Fort Worth to spend two days with Rod and Claudia. Ron was highly experienced in driving Volkswagens on icy streets and highways. It was a meaningful and joyful reunion, but Shelby was absent. Randall, Ron Alan, and Rhonda made it the first visit of these seven Stepps.

Christmas 1964, the Lee Roy Stepp family celebrated together again. They opened gifts at Daddy's home and enjoyed Mother's "hen and dressing" dinner. Shelby got his second record player, which was easier for him to use. The night before, all went to the apartment of Ron and Jeane with the Curfmans and watched seventeen-month-old Ron Alan open gifts with help from Steve.

In Fort Worth on New Year's Eve, Rod was calling on customers and stopped at AMSTAN-Plumbing, Heating & Air Conditioning, Sheet Metal. He had never heard of the business, but it was still open at 4:00 p.m., and he went in and gave Jack Futrell, the store manager, his M&M spiel, and left his business card and a M&M catalog.

On the following Tuesday, Rod picked up the M&M mail at the post office. As he was waiting at a stoplight noted for its long red-to-green interval, he thumbed through the mail and found an envelope from AMSTAN. As he opened it, he expected to see a request for additional information about a M&M product, but it was a purchase order for products that totaled $1,100. M&M had never received a PO for more than $300. Rod stepped out of his car and yelled a loud, "Whoopee." Today Rod still says it was probably his most exciting moment at M&M. The following year, AMSTAN was the largest customer of M&M, and they remained a valuable customer for many, many years.

In the *Burkburnett News* on January 12, 1965, was an article titled "Think You Got Troubles" that read as follows:

> Supposing you came into this world, minus hands and feet, left to a life with mere stubs to walk on,. arms that end in wrists...could you learn to walk, learn to play tunes on the piano? (This seems impossible, till you see it.) Opportunity Workshop in Wichita Falls has among its workers a little fellow who is in this condition, and he is one of the best workers in the shop.

The primary occupation at the Opportunity Workshop during the holidays was the making of stick-on type Christmas bows and candy wreaths.

Joe Hallford shared the following with Ronnie sometime in the 1980s:

> "Right after I got out of the Marines in 1965, I was working in Wichita Falls and getting started in my adult life. I do not recall how this encounter occurred or where I met this guy, but he talked me into helping coach a baseball team in the Boys Club Little League. The team practiced at Sam Houston School where I had

practiced in 1955 while playing for the Little Eagles[7] in the YMCA Kid Baseball League. I told the guy that I was excited about helping coach the boys, but that I was concerned about having never coached anything. I vividly remember the guy saying, 'Oh don't worry, I'll be the coach and tell you what to do. All you need to do is be at the practices and games and help me with the boys.'

"After a couple days of practice, this guy showed up at the practice field with all the baseball gear and dumped it out near the backstop. Then he said that he had a big job and would not be able to stay for practice that afternoon. We never saw him or heard from him again!

"I was twenty-one years old and had never done anything like this in my life. I had about twenty of the neatest boys from the Sam Houston neighborhood and did the best I could. I remembered the Little Eagle practices on the same rocky red clay field. Shelby heard about my coaching a ball team and showed up one day. I was throwing batting practice, and those boys couldn't hit their butt with a bass fiddle. I was throwing as easy as I could, but they could not hit the ball. Finally, I stopped and talked to them about watching the ball and standing in the batter's box and meeting the ball with the bat while extending their front foot.

"Then I said, 'Y'all sit down over there, and I will show you what I am talking about. Shelby, get up there and hit a few.' Shelby grabbed a bat and stood in the batter's box, and he hit every ball I threw. I threw to him much harder than I had to the boys. Shelby became the assistant coach, and the boys began to hit the ball.

"We did not win a trophy, but we did win some games, and I could not have been prouder of a group of kids or Shelby. He and I had been able to help a bunch of good kids play ball, and I learned that anyone can be of service to others. It is not so much about expertise, but more about willingness to serve.

"Two of those boys were brothers, and they lost their young dad[8] that year to leukemia. I reached out to them and took them fishing a few times. Being dumped on turned into a great experience for me, and it became somewhat of a turning point in my life.

"I hope I never forget those days with Yod, Yonnie, and Shelby."

In late May 1965 Jim Stepp graduated from Texas A&M. Steve finished fourth grade. Ron finished his courses and took two courses in summer school while working full-time. Ron enlisted players to make up a men's softball team at HHBC. He could not enlist a pitcher, so after playing shortstop for thirteen years he hurriedly learned to be a fast-pitch softball pitcher. Jerry Allen played third base and three of his brothers also played, and Shelby was the batboy. They did not win the league championship, but they won all but two of their league games and had a good time. Jerry and Rita became members of HHBC, attended regularly, served where they were needed, and Jerry later became an ordained deacon.

Shelby wrote Rod the following letter dated November 5, 1965:

Dear Rod, I am writing this letter to you for the sole purpose of answering the remarks you made about me going to a night club. I learned of this from your mother the other night while visiting and was a little disturbed about it.

I have gone to this one nightclub called the Ponderosa about five times for one reason—and one reason only—and that was merely to sit and listen to live music from a rock and roll band. I do not indulge in any alcoholic beverages or sit at the same table with people who do. Therefore, I strongly feel that my hands are clean.

I'm going all out to make up for everything I missed in my younger years. You might say my wild oats are being sown late in life.

I remember having to sit at home day in and day out while you and Ron went out and had a blast. It really didn't bother me that much, but I wanted to mention it just to put you to thinking how lucky it is for a person to be physically normal and be able to do things you did.

Let's go back to your college days at dear "ole panty wanty" A&M. Whenever parties were thrown, beer was always served. Of course, I know that you didn't take the stuff, but you were there. Being at those parties, were you condoning sin? That is about what you are saying I am doing.

Thus, there is no difference in me going to a nightclub and you going to those beer drinking parties.

May I kindly suggest that the next time you want to bark, make sure it is up the right tree!

Your cousin, Shelby Stepp

Note: When Ron started writing Shelby's story, he sent a questionnaire to about fifteen family members and friends of Shelby. Joe Hallford was one of the first to respond, and he also sent an article about Shelby that one of his friends submitted to him. The friend chose to be anonymous, but he unknowingly gave a comprehensive, interesting, and entertaining rebuttal to Rod's accusations of Shelby. Knowing Shelby as well as Ron does, as he read the article, his mind was presented with a motion picture of every movement of Shelby. Although the two evening events at the Ponderosa were about fifteen years apart, they are part of the same segment of Shelby's story. Ron takes this opportunity to thank the person who provided the *gem* that follows:

> Imagine if you will…you can close your eyes if that will help you imagine…
>
> You're in a honkytonk in Wichita Falls. Let's call it the Ponderosa after the popular family TV show of the times.
>
> Its over fifty years ago…and you are there…
>
> As you walk in you are met by the whaling sounds of the country and western band playing before a large group of appreciative revelers.
>
> Inside, the dance floor is crowded, and the air is smoky. Patrons not dancing are seated at various tables surrounding the large dance floor. Some rectangular tables are pushed together for large groups and some smaller round tables for couples or a small group. All appear to be having fun. Many are drinking beer and a lot are smoking cigarettes. At a lone table away from the dance floor is a man sitting by himself. He has a bottle of Coca-Cola in front of him and he is keeping time with the music by tapping the tabletop with his arm. You can see the man is handicapped. It appears he has no feet and no hands. In fact, one arm stops just below the elbow. The other, or right one, extends to where one's wrist would be.
>
> It is clear he is enjoying the music as he taps his shoes on the floor and his arms on the table. His shoes are simply tubular leather sleeves that lace up his legs with round leather soles. As you see him keeping time with the music, it is apparent he has talent for music and is immersed in

the moment. As the song ends, he applauds by clapping his two arms together as he enthusiastically nods his head in approval and appreciation.

The audience applauds as participants exit while others enter the dance floor. Thus, begins another song and no matter what it is…whether fast or slow, the man continues to listen and sip his coke all the while swaying with the music. After a while it is easy to see this young man is probably enjoying himself more than anyone else in the place. As the evening wears on the effect of the alcohol begins to take a toll on some of the partiers. It affects each differently, some become happy, others romantic, and some become belligerent, the man remains the same. Can you see him?

The music plays on.

Throughout the evening several people drop by and speak to the man. Many don't know him, but they have seen him around town and they just want to meet him and say hello. Due to the loud music and the man lacking a tongue some people have difficulty understanding his words, but the happy gestures and handshakes make up for it. The man not having a hand does not deter him from extending his right arm to acknowledge the greetings and well wishes of others. Even occasional slaps on the back were exchanged.

The young man's demeanor doesn't change as he continues to enjoy the music and sip his coke. Occasionally he will even get up and join in the dancing near the edge of the dance floor. On a couple of occasions some lady would join him as he danced. On those occasions after each dance, he would place his right arm across his waist and bend in a bow to the person as a way of saying thank you. Graciously he would return to his table for a sip of coke. You can see him, can't you?

During the course of the evening, this might repeat itself yet always it was a gracious exchange between two people enjoying themselves while immersed in the rhythm of music. And always the young man graciously bowed and applauded in appreciation. A true gentleman was he.

Before the hour became too late, he would finish off his coke (sometimes a second one) and make his exit with music in his heart and a smile on his face. Leaving everyone else to their own devices, he would have achieved what he intended…to enjoy a night of music in a happy atmosphere with a lot of happy people.

He never compromised his principles or values. The man was a witness wherever he walked…or danced.

You can open your eyes now. Celebrate Shelby, the gracious gentleman!

Anonymous
April 23, 2020

David Stepp became an M&M Manufacturing employee in the Wichita Falls plant on October 13, 1965.

In November of 1965, Roger Bacon and Ron went to Houston, Texas, to interview for jobs after they would graduate in late January of 1966. Ron interviewed for a computer programmer position at Texaco, Shell, and Gulf.

When the L. R. Stepp family celebrated Christmas on December 25, 1965, they knew that it would likely be the last one with Ron and Jeane living in Wichita Falls. That made this one dearer to the family. Mother cooked their favorite Christmas dinner again, gifts were opened and enjoyed, and the family visited for hours.

At the end of 1965, Shelby daily ate three meals, did his physical exercises, read the newspaper, listened to his transistor radio, watched TV, rode his adult tricycle, and practiced playing his marimba. Weekly, he worked weekdays at Opportunity Workshop, went to church on Sundays and Wednesdays, visited in five or six homes of family and friends, went to a movie theater, played a marimba solo at church or elsewhere, went to one or two ballgame(s), read all or part of a book, and wrote a letter. Shelby was happy with his life. He had lots of friends and a loving family including parents, brothers, aunts, uncles, and cousins. He was gratified that church members appreciated his service to God by playing his marimba in church services. *He kept on doing the best he could with what he had to the glory of God.*

Roger and Ron received job offers from Houston Belt and Terminal Railway and Gulf Oil in Houston, respectively. They both accepted their offer. After Midwestern State University graduation in late January, both families moved to the same apartment complex in Spring Branch in Houston in early February and began their new jobs.

Shelby and Ron would only see each other two or three times each year for the rest of Shelby's life. Ron's family always visited the Stepps and Curfmans in Wichita Falls at Christmas and usually twice each year at other times. Lee Roy, Stella, Shelby, and Steve visited them in Houston three times. Ron and Shelby only talked on the phone together once or twice each year, and they corresponded by mail with about the same frequency. Shelby always had a full schedule of work, church, visiting family and friends, etc. Ron and Jeane got even more involved at church, and they enjoyed seeing the popular sites in the Houston and surrounding areas. Ron was a computer programmer and often worked overtime on an urgent oil and gas production project after only six months at Gulf Oil. Ron and Jeane joined Clay Road Baptist Church (CRBC) in March 1966, and Jeane became church pianist within three months. Both began teaching Sunday school classes in 1967. Ron was ordained as a deacon in 1968 and began serving at that time. In later years, he became manager of a large group of computer systems analysts and programmers at Gulf Oil.

Rita Allen shared a summary of the four-decade friendship that she and Jerry had with Shelby:

> In the year 1964 my husband Jerry and I moved across the street from the Stepp family. That was the first time I saw Shelby Stepp. He had an adult tricycle (trike) that he rode everywhere. I was so fascinated and amazed at his ability to walk and ride with his severe disabilities.
>
> Jerry and I joined the same church that Shelby attended. Jerry joined the church's men's fast-pitch softball team. Shelby was the batboy for the team. He would run so fast to take care of the bats and was such an inspiration to me, and to everyone else I am sure.
>
> We moved about a mile away from Shelby a couple of years later. He would ride his trike over to our house often to visit. On Sunday nights after church, we usually ate hot dogs. Jerry would chop them up real fine for Shelby, so he was able to eat one.
>
> Often Jerry would go pick Shelby up and take him to ball games and other places. Shelby liked to watch Midwestern State University men's basketball games and WFSH football and basketball games.
>
> One year we took Shelby to a Texas Ranger game in Arlington, Texas. He loved the Dodgers and wore his Dodger shirt and cap. Jerry teased him a lot, which Shelby liked. Jerry coached boy's baseball teams for years and Shelby was his batboy. Jerry loved and admired Shelby and enjoyed taking him places. I am sure that Jerry[9] would have lots of things to tell you about him.
>
> Shelby was in a bowling league at Village Bowl[10] He was a man of many talents and often

played his marimba for our church and many other churches. I loved to hear and watch him play "The King Is Coming" when he would almost dance around while playing. Shelby loved the Lord Jesus, and it was evident in his life. I think his greatest handicap was his speech impediment. Shelby made up for it in his actions.

In May 1968, Jim Stepp had completed eighteen of his twenty-seven months to earn a law degree. He suddenly decided that he did not want to be a lawyer, and he just quit. He had always wanted to own a small grocery store, but he went to work at M&M in Fort Worth to earn enough money to buy and operate a grocery store. He took care of the bookkeeping and other business accounting matters.

Jeane's grandmother, Ida Pearl Curfman, died on June 3, 1969, at the age of eighty-two. She was buried in Rosemont Cemetery. She was a hardworking Christian woman.

As the 1960s became history, Shelby became more aware that he would always be limited in job opportunities because of his speech impediment. Even with the training in speech that he was taught and trained to use by Mrs. Lucas, only a few could always understand what Shelby said. Mother, Mrs. Lucas, Ronnie, Uncle Ike, Jerry and Rita Allen, David, Aunt Ruby, Aunt Lydia, Rod, Butch, and Jim Stepp were about all who could. And most all jobs where speech was not an issue required manual labor that Shelby could not physically do.

When his job at Opportunity Workshop ceased to meet his income requirements,[11] Shelby was hired by Highland Heights Baptist Church in 1970 as assistant custodian.

At that time, Ron was taken aback by this development in Shelby's life. Ron's thinking was, "Is this all there is for Shelby who overcame unequaled disabilities, earned high school and business college diplomas, was blessed with a sharp mind, had a good work ethic, loved people and had many friends, had a deep faith in God, and never gave in to despair?"

Twenty-two years passed before Ron realized the positive impact that Shelby had on people's lives from 1945 to 1992 without making a single public speech. And in 2005, after Shelby's death, Ron came to fully realize the scope of Shelby's life of inspiration as an incredible boy who was the personification of *The Little Engine That Could*[12] and a remarkable man who was "a man of few words." Humanly speaking, Shelby's most severe handicap was his speech impairment. But in God's plan, Shelby's inspiring life spoke more loudly and more effectively than any conversations or speeches could ever have achieved.

At the beginning of Shelby's custodial work at HHBC in 1970, he could sweep floors and sidewalks; dust pianos, furniture, and shelves; pick up Sunday bulletins; replace hymnals in the pew racks; etc. Over the following twenty-six years, his duties increased as described in entries taken from his partial diary of 1987 in the next chapter and from his partial diary of 1996 in chapter 7. Many HHBC members came and went during those years, and many of them commented positively about Shelby's work ethic.

In 1972, Steve was riding in the back seat of a jeep with three buddies from WF on a gravel road at Possum Kingdom Lake when the jeep turned over. All four were injured and were taken to the closest hospital in Graham, Texas. Immediate attention was given to a boy that had head wounds. After a while, Steve was attended to, and it was soon determined that he had life-threatening internal injuries. He had almost bled to death at that point. Mother and Daddy were called and informed of Steve's condition. Mother immediately drove to Graham to be with Steve while surgery on his ruptured liver was performed. Mother called Ron at his home in Houston.

Ron, Jeane, and Ron Alan arrived at the hospital about five hours later. Steve's surgery went well, but he would require additional surgery while his buddies would be released the next day. When informed that Steve would be transferred to a Dallas hospital for the second surgery, Mother decided to go with him and stay at the hospital until he was released. Ron, Jeane, and Ron Alan went to Wichita Falls to pick up Shelby and take him to Houston to stay until Mother could return home.

After packing Shelby's clothes, shaving kit, etc., and marimba in their large station wagon, Ron drove 385 miles to his home in northwest Houston. Although Jeane and Ron knew much about what Shelby liked to eat and how food needed to be specially prepared, there were times when he was not satisfied with his meal. Shelby never hesitated to make his wishes known, which was no surprise to Jeane and Ron. They had seen similar exchanges between Shelby and Mother.

The first morning, Shelby complained that he needed a larger bowl for his cereal and an extra spoon. He said that he would not reuse his cereal spoon to eat his baby food. The next morning when he came to his place at the table, he saw a large mixing bowl and a line of eight spoons next to the bowl that Ron had placed there. He stood by his chair, gazed at the bowl and spoons, put his right stub on the back of his head, turned and looked at Ron and Jeane, and gave them his "famous grin."

Shelby went with Ron's family to Sunday school, Sunday worship services both morning and night, and Wednesday night prayer service at Clay Road Baptist Church (CRBC). Ron arranged for Shelby to play his marimba and demonstrate some of his athletic prowess at one of the Wednesday night prayer meetings. Shelby was a big hit with all ages that night.

Mother called to say that Steve's second surgery went well in Parkland Memorial Hospital, the same Dallas hospital where President Kennedy had died. The surgeon was surprised to find a sponge had been left in Steve's abdomen when he was sewed up after his first surgery was done. One year later, Steve had the highest score in the physical fitness test in his US Army Basic Combat Training unit.

One afternoon the Stepp foursome went to the Astrodome to see the Houston Astros play the Los Angeles Dodgers. Shelby wore his LA Dodger T-shirt and cap. His favorite pitcher, Sandy Koufax, shut out the Astros, and the Dodgers won 3–0. Shelby hollered often, jumped out of his seat several times, and took off his cap and saluted several Dodger players when they did something outstanding. Astros fans around him seemed to appreciate Shelby's visible support of his Dodgers.

Shelby enjoyed staying with Ron, Jeane, and nine-year-old Ron Alan, but he missed his family and friends in Wichita Falls, working at HHBC, riding his trike, and more. After six or seven weeks, Shelby got to go back home.

Harry S. Ewing died in 1974 at the age of forty-one. He was the first person to be buried in one of Daddy's six gravesites.

Rafael Cruz became a Christian at CRBC in 1975 when his son Ted was age four. During their years at CRBC, Rafael always referred to Ted as "Felito." Jeane was Felito's teacher in first grade Sunday school and his leader in Children's choir for several years. He was a bright student and a super active boy. Ted became a Christian at age eight in 1979 at CRBC. He later became US Senator from Texas on January 3, 2013. Shelby did not visit Ron in Houston during the six years that the Cruz family were members at CRBC. Neither Rafael nor Ted ever got to meet Shelby. They both would have enjoyed him.

In December 1979, Ron and Jeane hosted a party for Daddy's seventy-fifth birthday. They sent invitations to family and friends in November. Ron made an album with photos of Daddy from 1933 to 1975 to give to Daddy at the birthday party. Thirty-one family and friends attended his party at HHBC.

Uncle Johna Ewing died on February 27, 1981, at the age of seventy-four.

Uncle Sonny Stepp died on October 24, 1981, at the age of seventy-two. Shelby and Ron lost their favorite uncle. He was buried in Greenwood Memorial Park in Fort Worth.

Uncle Charles M. Vernon died on April 11, 1982, at the age of ninety. He was married to Aunt Sally Stepp.

Aunt Era May Stepp Bond died on February 10, 1983, at the age of eighty-one.

David had bought a 1957 Chevy Bel Air sedan in 1977, and he had the original 283 V8 motor rebuilt in 1981 by Al Weiss who was a mechanic for Eddie Hill during some of his world championship years in drag racing. It was turquoise on bottom and white on top. David got his buddy Glen McShan to repaint it black. Then he got family friend Melvin Weatherford to reupholster the interior with red Naugahyde and install red carpet in the floorboard. Finally, he had red pinstriping added. Ron bought the car from David in the summer of 1983 for $4,000 and drove it home to Jersey Village. Ron gave the car to Brandon in 2017. In 2021, the car would sell for $27,000 to $30,000.

Uncle John E. Stepp died on December 11, 1983, at the age of eighty. He was buried at Shoat Springs Cemetery east of Hugo, Oklahoma.

Jeane's dad, Wilburn "Webb" Arthur Curfman, died on December 14, 1983, at the age of sixty-nine. Reverend Jim McCurley officiated the service. Webb was revered by the Ron Stepp family, and Ron often said he was the best line drive hitter that he ever played with or against in fast-pitch softball.

In 1984, Village Seven Presbyterian in Colorado Springs, Colorado, invited Shelby to play his marimba at their annual Music Evangelism Foundation Bible Conference. They stated that his travel expenses would be reimbursed. A couple from HHBC graciously took him to the event. The roundtrip was almost 1,200 miles. After playing his marimba, Shelby received a standing ovation from the audience of about 2,500. His concert was so entertaining that he was invited again the following year. In 1985, the same couple took Shelby again, and the same size audience gave him the same standing ovation. Shelby was invited again many years, but he could not get the transportation and special care that he required.

On April 8, 1986, Shelby celebrated his fiftieth birthday at home with many family members and friends. Rod, Butch, and Jim gave him his first TV. As always, Shelby's greatest joy came from being with large groups of family and friends. He ended his fiftieth year with a positive attitude about his work and service at HHBC, his loving family life, his many friends, and his private life, but he was not content being without a female companion.

* * * * *

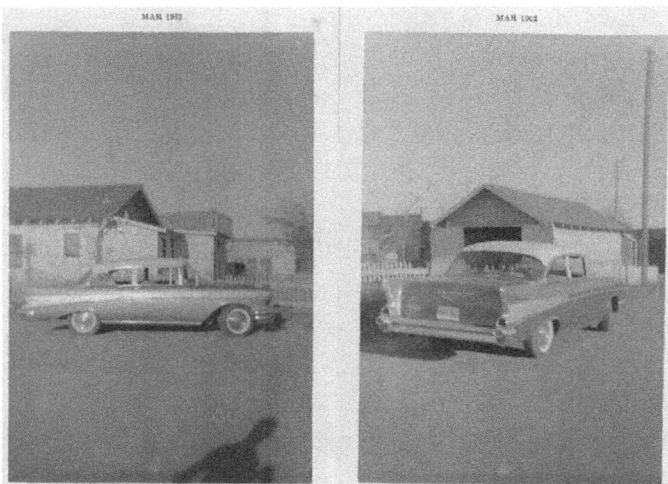

This 1957 Chevrolet Bel Air is the only road vehicle that Shelby ever drove. His home is in the background. The car is parked on the HHBC parking lot in 1962.

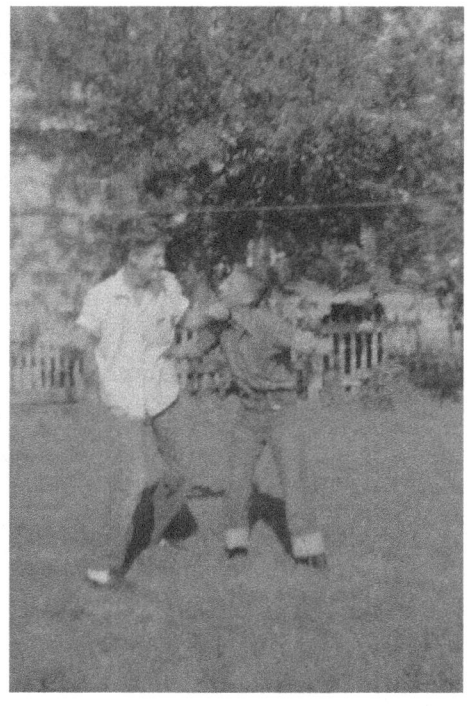

Shelby and Cousin Dennis Mansell in a playful slugfest in March 1962

AN INCREDIBLE BOY AND A REMARKABLE MAN

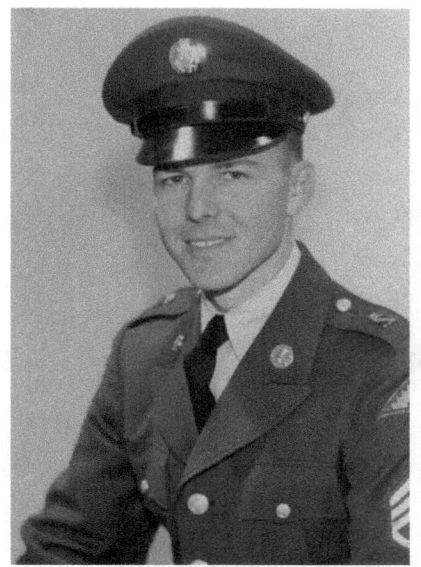

Staff Sergeant Stepp in November 1962

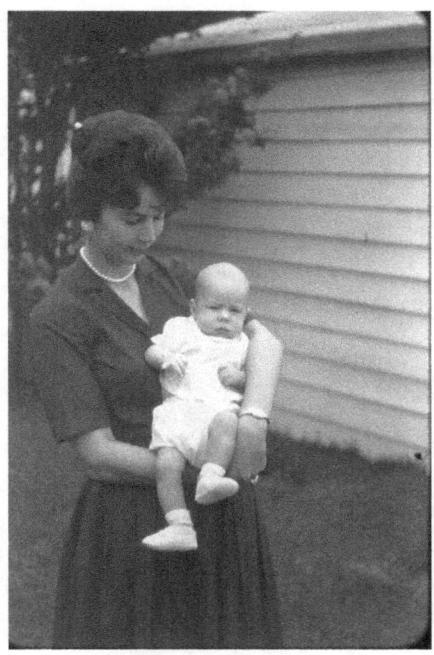

Jeane with Shelby's first nephew, Ron Alan, in 1963.

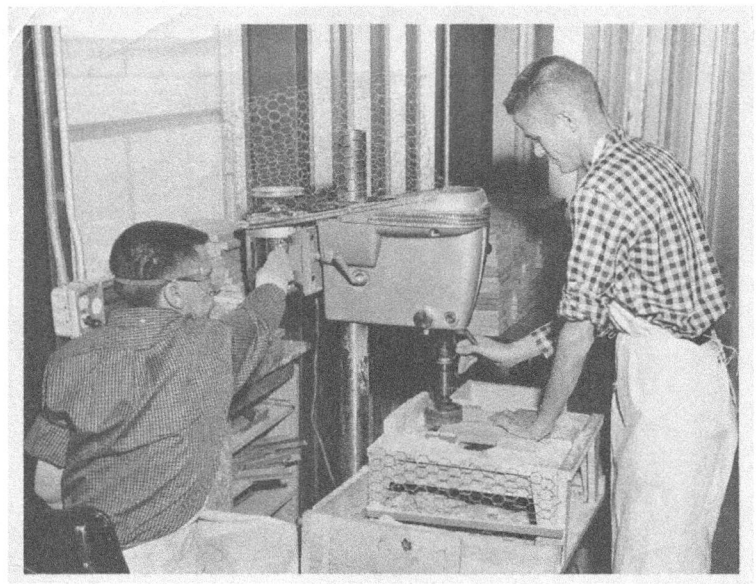

Shelby and co-worker at Opportunity Workshop in 1964

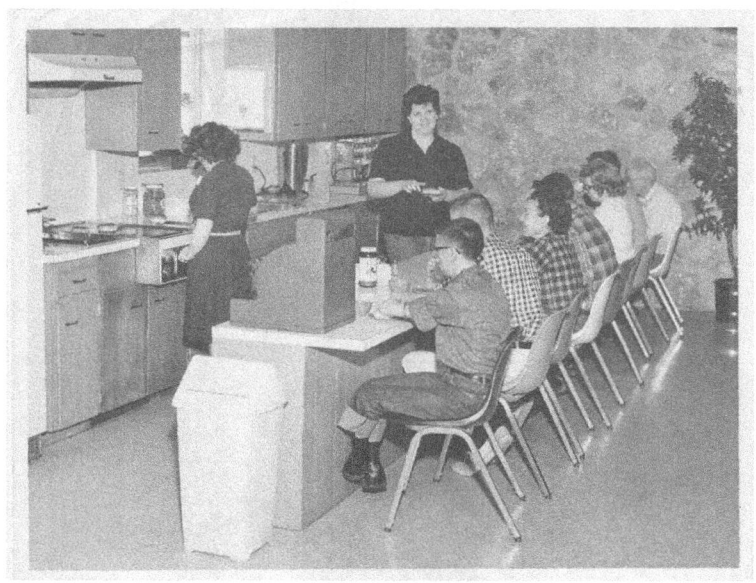

Shelby and co-workers during lunch break in 1964

AN INCREDIBLE BOY AND A REMARKABLE MAN

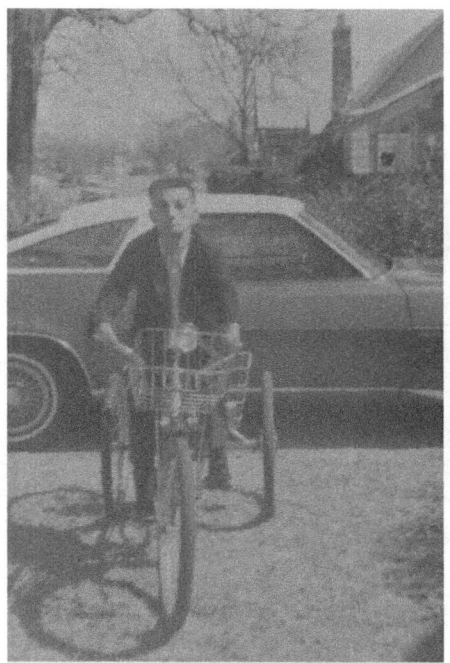

Shelby on his first trike in 1975

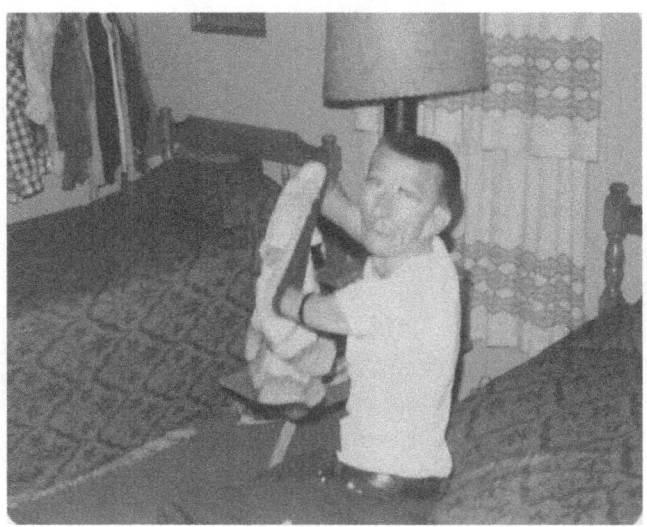

Shelby putting on his favorite style shirt in 1983.
It is a slip-over with no buttons.

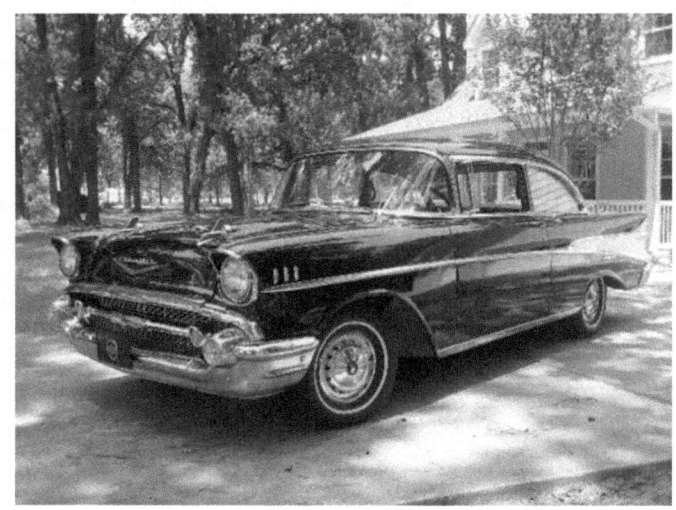

Ron's '57 Chevy that he bought from David in 1983.

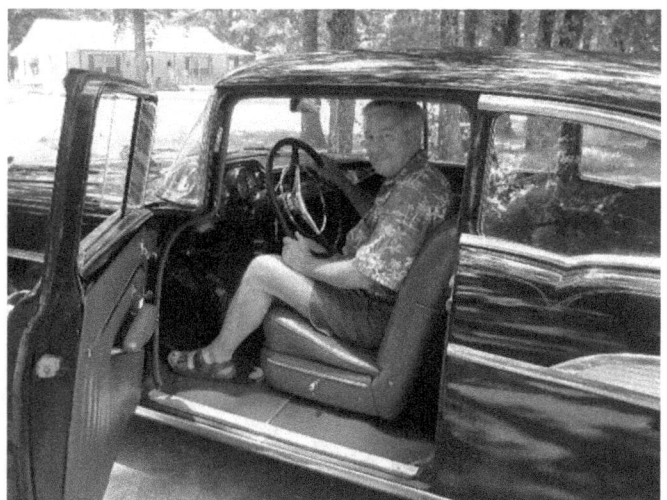

Ron gave it to Brandon in 2017.

AN INCREDIBLE BOY AND A REMARKABLE MAN

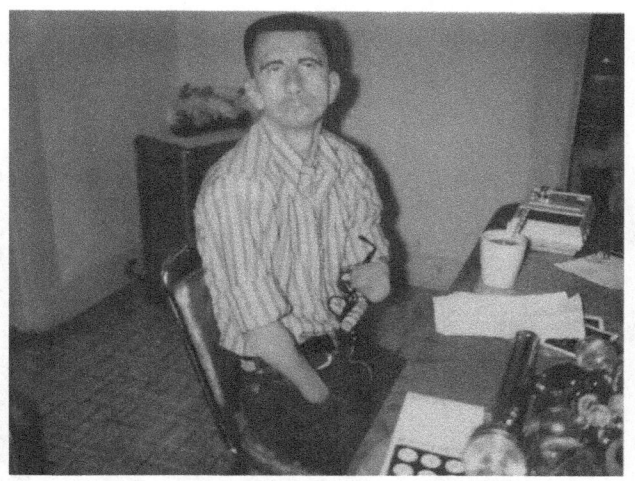

Shelby in his office at HHBC in 1985

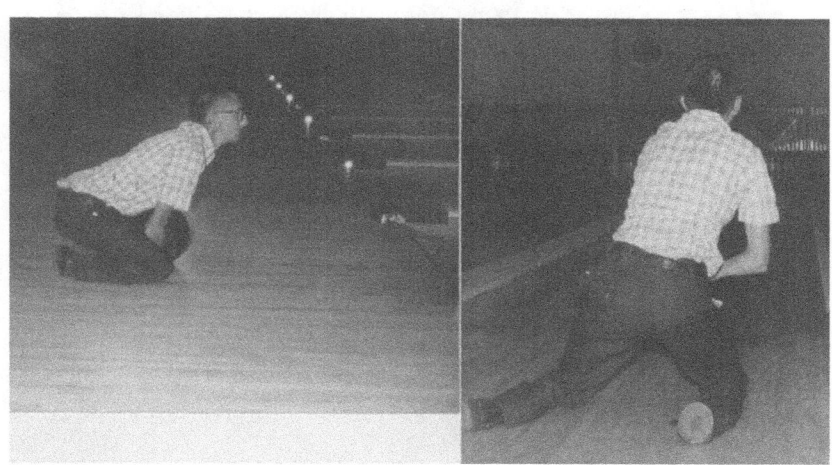

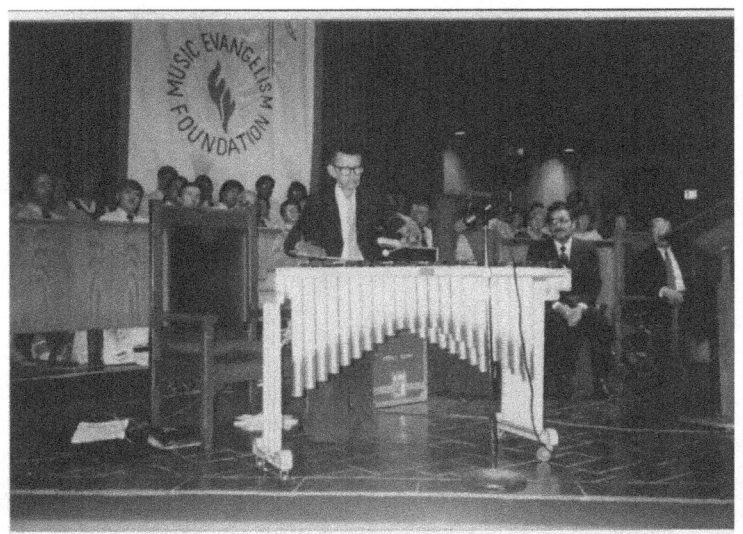

This photo was taken in 1985 of Shelby playing his marimba at the Music Evangelism Foundation Bible Conference in Colorado Springs, Colorado, before an audience of about 2,500. He received a standing ovation. Executive Director Jamall Badry is seated to his left with his hands together. Shelby had played there in 1984 and would play there again in 2002.

AN INCREDIBLE BOY AND A REMARKABLE MAN

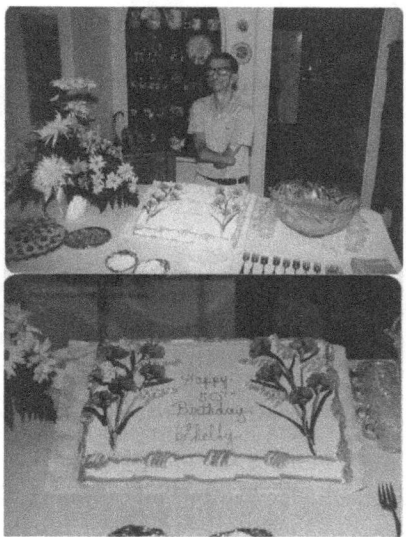

Shelby's 50th birthday on April 8, 1986 at Daddy's and Mother's house. About 30 family and friends attended.

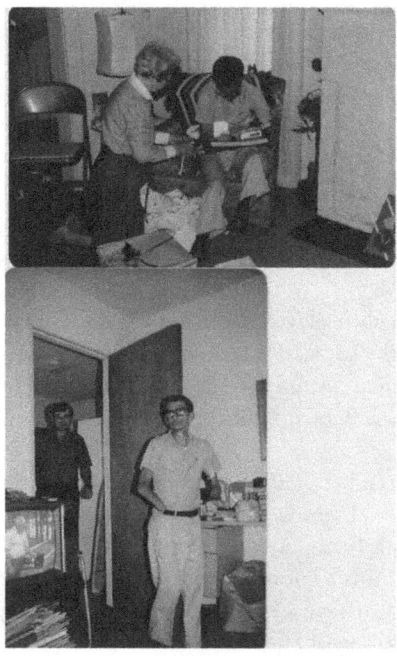

Top: Mother helps Shelby open gifts. Bottom: Butch shows Shelby his first personal TV.

1. The Sozialistische Einheitspartei Deutschlands (SED) was founded on April 21, 1946, by a merger of the Social Democratic Party of Germany (SPD) and the Communist Party of Germany (KPD), which was based in the Soviet-occupation zone of Germany and the Soviet-occupied sector of Berlin. It was dissolved on December 16, 1989.
2. East Germany, officially the German Democratic Republic, was a country that existed from 1949 to 1990.
3. *Jet* is an American weekly magazine that focuses on news, culture, and entertainment related to the African American community. Founded in November 1951 by John H. Johnson of the Johnson Publishing Company in Chicago, Illinois, the magazine was initially billed as "The Weekly Negro News Magazine." *Jet* chronicled the Civil Rights Movement from its earliest years, including the murder of Emmett Till, the Montgomery bus boycott, and the activities of Civil Rights leader Martin Luther King Jr. The *Jet* issue with an article about Shelby was in 1960. A Google search found all weekly issues from 1955 to 1963 except those from April 28 to October 20 of 1960. By deduction, the issue with Shelby on the cover was in that missing period. It was a very disappointing search for Ron. All the covers from 1955 to 1963 featured only Blacks, which makes the issue with Shelby's article most unique.

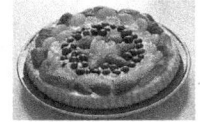

4. Frau Albert's German fruitcakes 1960–62.
5. As of April 8, 2021, Ron has not smoked a cigarette, cigar, or pipe since February 5, 1963, nor has he used any product to assist him in breaking the habit of smoking.
6. Mother always preferred a large hen to a turkey.
7. David Stepp played centerfield for the Little Eagles in 1955, and they were City Champions of the YMCA Kid Baseball Midget League. Joe Hallford also played on that team.
8. In 1963 and 1964, Ron played shortstop on the Downtown Baptist Church softball team. Dwight Ledford was their pitching ace and was the dad of those two boys. Dwight died on August 18, 1965. Ron and Jeane went to Dwight's funeral at Downtown Baptist Church. He was a good, Godly man, who gave Ron wise counsel.
9. Jerry Allen died December 5, 2010. At the time of his death, he was the beloved coach of the volleyball teams at Wichita Christian School. He started club volleyball in Wichita Falls and coached hundreds of girls for thirty-six years. In prior years, Jerry was a vocational education teacher in WFISD and taught auto body repair at Carrigan Center. Ron regrets that Jerry Allen did not live to contribute to the writing of Shelby's story.
10. Photos will show how Shelby bowled. His top score is unknown, but in a diary entry for February 25, 1996, he wrote, "My high game of the three games was

AN INCREDIBLE BOY AND A REMARKABLE MAN

a sizzling 141." Village Bowl was 1.7 miles from home. Shelby would get on his knees near the bowling lane facing the pins. A bowler would place Shelby's ball between his knees. Shelby would push the ball with both stubs. In 20 to 25 seconds the ball would hit the pins. He rarely guttered. His highest recorded score was 147.

[11] Shelby received a monthly disability pension check from Uncle Sam.

[12] *The Little Engine That Could* is an American folktale (existing in the form of several illustrated children's books and films) that became widely known in the

CHAPTER 7

Late Adult Years: Fifty-One to Sixty-Seven (1987–2003)

In 1987, Shelby had worked as assistant custodian at HHBC for seventeen years. He had become more proficient in performing those duties that he was still doing, and he had been assigned additional duties during those years. The following entries from his partial diary of early 1987 inform the reader of his custodial work at HHBC, his relationships with family and friends, his recreational life, and his service to God.

> Like New Year's Day in the past I awakened this morning to flip on the tube to watch the Cotton Bowl and Rose Bowl Parades. I went to Village Bowl this afternoon and whiled the time away bowling four games. My high game was 120. (Thursday, January 1, 1987).
>
> I started off the first Saturday of the new year at the downtown YMCA. I sat and read the newspaper along with listening to a basketball game on my transistor radio. In the evening I went to see Mutt and Ruby McShan. (Saturday, January 3)

AN INCREDIBLE BOY AND A REMARKABLE MAN

On most Saturdays, Shelby went to the YMCA downtown and spent three or four hours reading and listening to sports on his transistor radio, which aired the audio of TV channels. Mostly he watched on TV or listened to college and professional football and basketball and major league baseball. One of the caretakers provided his transportation. He still rode his trike often but usually for less than four miles.

> This afternoon I wheeled over to Louis's and Lydia's to visit. Louis and I watched the NFL playoff game between the New York Giants and the San Francisco 49'ers. (Sunday, January 4)
>
> The Ewing Bible Study resumed today after taking the Christmas and New Year break. The study was held at Aunt Ruth Erwin's apartment at Midtown Manor. Bud started a new series in the Book of Matthew. (Tuesday, January 6)
>
> At work I got outside a little while after lunch to sweep off the porch and sidewalk behind the Sanctuary and grass and debris along the sidewalk. Then I wound it up going around the entire church lawn and the parking lot across the street. (Wednesday, January 7)
>
> Tonight was my first visit of the new year to Ruby's and J. D.'s. They expressed again to me their appreciation for the Halley's Bible Commentary books I had given for Christmas. They said the books really help them in teaching the Sunday School lessons. (January 8)
>
> This evening I made another visit to Mutt and Ruby McShan's home. (January 9)
>
> It was back to the "Y" today for my regular Saturday visit there. (January 10)
>
> I made a return Sunday afternoon visit to Louis's and Lydia's. We talked about what each

other had done during the week. There were two NFL games today. (January 11)

Glenn Wilson and his wife Ernestine, who are very good friends and former members of HHBC, were very gracious to let me into their home this evening. We had a real good visit as usual. (January 12)

Mother's illness kept her from going to the Ewing Bible Study. Aunt Sis and Jimmy came by to pick me up to go to the Bible study at Uncle Tommy's and Aunt Nila's. (January 13)

I spent most of the day outdoors at work raking up some more leaves. (January 14)

I went over to see Chester and Faye Hallford tonight. (January 15)

I ran into a pretty good size job in the Sanctuary scrubbing up black marks made by shoes on the floor tiles in between the pews. I used a new kind of soap, that Glenn Harper (Custodian) bought last month, and Comet to scrub with steel wool. (Tuesday, January 20)

I worked on the north side of the Sanctuary until noon cleaning up skid marks between the pews. I had to stop to vacuum the carpet to prepare for tonight's midweek service. (January 21)

I worked upstairs most of the day scrubbing skid marks off the floor in the two restrooms, the kitchen, and the adjacent hallway going to the men's room. I got that much done around 3:00 p.m. This evening I pedaled my 3-wheeler over to Louis's and Lydia's. (January 23)

After having to stay home last week because of the snow and ice, I got to go down to the YMCA for my Saturday visit. I did the usual of reading the paper and listening to some college basketball on my transistor radio. (January 24)

I took one of my bowling balls out to Village Bowl. I bowled three games and had a high game of 109. [He should have taken his other ball.] I had to get back to church before Church Training [at 6:00 p.m.] to unlock the Sanctuary and turn up the heat Glenn had to go out of town. (January 25)

This evening I visited in the home of Virgil and Vivian Clark on Miami Street and had a good time with them. They are the sister and brother-in-law of Bobby Allred, a paraplegic who has become a very good friend of mine. Vivian invited me to Bobby's birthday party tomorrow! (Monday, January 26)

I attended Bobby's birthday party at the Heritage Manor where he lives. Vivian and Virgil were gracious to pick me up and take me with them. Bobby really had a big party. There were about 60 people there. Some square dancing was the entertainment. Bobby got lot of real nice gifts. (January 27)

I have just come home from visiting with Ruby and J. We had another good time together. (January 29)

I went to the Grant Street Park to sit on a picnic table bench to read and listen to some basketball. (January 30)

The nightly visiting this time took me to Chester's and Faye's. I was fortunate to find ole Faye in a good mood. The three of us had a good chit-chat. (January 31)

The Ewing Bible Study was held in our home this evening. The attendance was the best it has been in quite some time. There were 15 of us. (February 3)

> I began the big job of scrubbing black marks and wax off the tile floor upstairs in the long hallway of the Education Building. I got one-third of it done. It is a very tedious job. (February 4)
>
> I made about an equal amount of progress as yesterday on the cleaning job on the tile floor upstairs. This evening I made another of my regular Thursday night visits with Ruby and J. D. I took some cookies of several different flavors and we ate them along with drinks. Ruby and J. drank Dr Pepper and I drank coffee. (February 7, 1987)

The rest of Shelby's 1987 diary is not available, if it ever existed. Shelby later made entries in that same diary book starting with February 8, 1996.

Uncle Willie L. "Bud" Ewing died in August of 1987 at the age of sixty-one.

Four days before Christmas of 1987, while Shelby was at a friend's house watching a Dallas Cowboy football game, his specially designed three-wheeler was stolen. The following are excerpts from an article in the *Wichita Daily Times* on January 4, 1988:

> A man who knew Stepp casually from times when the 51-year-old church janitor watched him play tennis has located a cycle that they plan to modify for Stepp. Denny Bishop, a city real estate agent, said the only real problems are replacing hand brakes with pedal-operated ones and adjusting the seat so Stepp will be able to reach the pedals.
>
> "We're going to get wheels back to Shelby," Bishop said.
>
> He said he first met Stepp when Stepp would pedal to the park [Hamilton Park] where Bishop played tennis. "It didn't seem to matter to

him whether it was a big tennis tournament or a little one. He'd always come up. I admired his spunk," Bishop said.

Stella Stepp said her son…had been pedaling the yellow Schwinn cycle across Wichita Falls for about 15 years after he bought it in the mid-70s with savings from $30-a-week paychecks. Stella Stepp said Bishop's offer was one of several that came for her son. "We appreciate everything that's been done," she said.

Aunt Velma Cody Stepp died on August 1, 1988, at the age of eighty-four. She was buried at Shoat Springs near Hugo, Oklahoma.

Ron and Jeane were blessed with a grandson on March 2, 1990. He was named Brandon Alan Stepp. A few weeks later, Jeane began caring for him Monday through Friday.

At the age of eighty-seven, Daddy was diagnosed with colon cancer and had successful surgery.

Ron and Jeane became grandparents again. Brittany Lynn Stepp was born on June 11, 1992. Ron retired from Chevron in September of 1992. They enjoyed caring for Brandon and Brittany for several years.

J. D. Faulkenberry died at the age of sixty-eight on December 8, 1992, in Wichita Falls, Texas.

Daddy, Mother, and Shelby visited Ron's family in Jersey Village at Christmas in 1992. Ron had asked them to bring Shelby's marimba, mallets, music stand, and music to play a concert at Houston Northwest Baptist Church, Ron's church. Ron then arranged with Pastor Bill Bennett and Minister of Music Dan St. Andre for Shelby to be featured in a Sunday evening worship service.

At the beginning of the service, Ron introduced Shelby and read his biography[1] including his salvation experience.[2] Shelby then performed an inspiring thirty-five-minute marimba concert accompanied by Jeane on the piano. The audience of about five hundred gave them a standing ovation at the end. Daddy and Mother sat on the front row along with Ron Alan, his wife, and two-year-old

Brandon. Ron sat between Ron Alan and Daddy and was impressed by the look of astonishment on Daddy's face. It was obvious to Ron that Daddy had never witnessed that kind of response to Shelby's playing his marimba.

After returning home, Shelby wrote the following in a letter to Ron:

> I still haven't gotten over the great response the Northwest Baptist Church gave me in my musical performance. It touched me deeply. Give to Dan, your music director, my thanks for permitting me the opportunity to give my testimony in music. And of course, giving credit where credit is due, thanks to you for the splendid job of presenting my biography, and to Jeane for her superb job of accompanying me on the piano.
>
> Tell Brandon that Bubba said hello.
>
> Love, Shelby

In August 1993, Jim Stepp had been employed at M&M for twenty-five years, and he retired when he turned fifty. He had always stated that he would retire at age fifty.

Aunt Imogene Randolph Ewing had Alzheimer's disease in her last years, and Uncle Ike treated her like his little girl. He kept her well-dressed with her hair always looking pretty. She died on January 2, 1994, at the age of eighty-two.

In early 1994, it became apparent to Ron that Mother and Daddy required twenty-four-hour care. Mother was not able to do much physically because of increasingly poor heart function, and Daddy's dementia was worsening. He discussed the issue with his brothers and soon hired three women through an agency to work eight-hour shifts to prepare meals, keep house, provide transportation, buy groceries, and give additional care for Daddy, Mother, and Shelby as needed. The caregivers were Debbie Neinas, Gladys Foster, and Lou Anne. Ron was required to handle the bookkeeping and filing reports for household employees required by government agencies. Good care was provided by the caretakers for the thirty months they were employed, but the cost averaged $90,000 per year.

Uncle Thomas L. Ewing died on April 3, 1994, one day before his eighty-sixth birthday.

Shelby celebrated his fifty-eighth birthday on April 8.

For Ron's fifty-seventh birthday on May 1, 1994, Shelby wrote the following in a letter:

> Ron, I remember those days of our childhood when we used to play cowboys and Indians. At times when we'd go see those western movies and reenact some of the scenes after getting home. Yes, there were some good serials we saw on Saturday afternoons when we lived in Hugo, Oklahoma, and back in Wichita Falls.
>
> I can just remember three of them. In Hugo there was one called "The Black Whip." It was about a young woman attired in black and used a whip for a weapon. Back in Wichita Falls, there was "Nyoka, the Jungle Girl" and "Jack Armstrong, All-American Boy." Oh yes, I forgot back in Hugo we got to see a western movie where we heard Sunset Carson "talk through his nose."
>
> I remember those days we had our fictitious high school and college teams. In high school I had the Vega Greyhounds and you (the) Northrop (Broncos).
>
> I remember how we would get out in the backyard and play out their games against other opponents and against each other. Yep, we became archrivals with those two teams and the real-life teams, the New York Yankees and Brooklyn Dodgers. It was appalling to me how those so-called Bronx Bombers could luck out

to win five of the 6 World Series from 1949 to 1954. The really best team, the Dodgers, won in 1955.

I just wanted to write to let you know that I haven't forgotten the good times we had together and want to express to you my warmest appreciation for taking the time to do the things mentioned above with me.

I am enclosing a check for $25.00 as a belated birthday gift. Happy 39th(?)

> Your loving brother,
> Shelby

In mid-May of 1994, Daddy, Mother, and Shelby visited Ron and Jeane in their home in Jersey Village. Mother especially wanted to visit her great-grandchildren Brandon and Brittany. It was an enjoyable three-day visit for all.

Ron got his first colonoscopy on May 27, 1994, and also had a polypectomy. Because he had polyps, though not cancerous like Daddy's, Ron began to encourage Shelby to have a colonoscopy.

Ron began employment as business manager at St. Christopher Episcopal Church in August 1994. Jeane continued caring for Brandon and Brittany.

Uncle Ike married Alma who was his neighbor and had helped Ike take care of Imogene after she was diagnosed with Alzheimer's disease.

In late 1995, Veronica was added to the team of caretakers.

Following are selected entries from Shelby's diary of 1996 beginning with February 8.

> After taking care of the Sanctuary this morning, vacuuming the carpet and sweeping between the pews, I went to the barber shop to get my ears lowered. (February 8, 1996) [Beginning in 1963, Shelby always got a flattop haircut.]

I worked in two areas today—the kitchen and my office, taking inventory of kitchen supplies, plastic bowls, and paper plates took up a lot of the time. I attended the last home game of the Notre Dame High's boy basketball team. [Shelby knew some of their players.] (February 9)

I went to Walmart and bought Mother a sweater and card for her birthday and a Valentine card. (February 10)

Today was Mother's birthday. She is now 82 years young. I presented her the sweater and birthday card. (Sunday, February 11)

The Women's Missionary Union (WMU) held its monthly meeting and luncheon. Mary Dawn Cantu, my late Uncle Bud's youngest daughter, gave a talk. Vivian Haney came to practice a couple of songs to play next Sunday. We decided on "I Saw the Light" and "The Healer." "Standing on a Solid Rock" was picked as an extra song. (February 12)

After cleaning the Young Adults classroom and the Fellowship Hall I went outdoors to rake leaves on the west side of the Education Building. I started after 10 a.m. and did not finish until a little after 2 p.m. The SS Adult Department had a Valentine's Banquet at Luby's Cafeteria. There were 48 attendees. I played "I Saw the Light" and "The Healer." (February 14)

On a beautiful fall-like day, I enjoyed watching some tennis matches at the Hamilton Park courts. Then I went to the "Y" as usual. In the evening hours I was at the D. L. Ligon Coliseum watching the MSU Indians men's basketball team play their final game of the season. They beat Tarleton State 90–86. (February 17)

At my request Bobby and Mary Byrd had coffee with me at Taco Bell. (February 21)

Clifford Irby and I watched a sequel to "Halloween 4" and "Outlaw Josey Wales" at "Irby's Theater." The latter starred Clint Eastwood, Sondra Locke, and Will Sampson. (February 22)

Another busy Friday. I started the day vacuuming the carpet in the auditorium; sweeping and mopping the floor in the foyer; cleaning baby beds, chest of drawers, and children rocking chair; polishing the big rocker; and vacuuming the rug. After lunch I cleaned the pastor's office and the other offices. I rode my trike to Sikes Senter Theater tonight to see "City Hall" starring Al Pacino. I then stopped at Taco Bell on Kemp Blvd to have coffee. (February 23)

This morning when Debbie came to my room to put my shoes on my feet, she said that Dad had another bad spell last night. Like three nights before, he stopped breathing for a little bit. After taking me to the "Y," Debbie took Dad to the hospital. The doctor put him on a different medicine. (Saturday, February 24)

I went to Village Bowl this afternoon to do some bowling. My high game of the three games was a sizzling 141. There was a spirit-filled "Singspiration" tonight. There were lots of good solos, duets, trios, and a piano/organ duet. I played "Where the Soul Never Dies" and "In the Shadow of the Cross." (February 25)

I worked most of the day up in the balcony of the Sanctuary, using Endust spray to clean the pews, stairway bannisters, table, PA system, and cassette player. I vacuumed the carpets in the balcony and stairsteps. This evening I got to see a

AN INCREDIBLE BOY AND A REMARKABLE MAN

movie that I have wanted to see for a long time. It was "In the Line of Fire" starring Clint Eastwood. He is after an assassin who plans to murder the president. Eastwood kills the would-be assassin. (February 27)

On the last working day of the week, I first took care of the offices and finished taking inventory of supplies. This afternoon I practiced on the 12 songs to be played at Monterey Care Center next Tuesday. I rode my trike to Bobby Evans Sporting Goods Store to buy some kneepads. Tonight, I went to Sikes Senter Theater to see "Rumble in the Bronx." I got stopped by a cop for not having lights on my trike. (March 1)

With the WMU scheduled to have a potluck supper in Fellowship Hall, I put trash bags in the two 33-gallon trash cans. I went back to church at 5:30 p.m. to open the Education Building and Sanctuary and turn on the heating. I took my supper and ate in my office. (Monday, March 4)

Another Saturday at the "Y" reading the newspaper and listening to some college basketball championship games. Ron and Jeane came to pick me up. At home I visited with them for an hour. (March 9)

This afternoon I triked out to Village Bowl to bowl three games. I had a pretty good day, especially the first game which was 149. I started that game like wildfire getting two spares and two strikes in the first four frames. (March 10)

Most all of my workday was taken up in the kitchen scrubbing the sink, shelves, stove, microwave, lunch trays, and refrigerator. Then I swept and mopped the floors. (March 12)

I am most upset at the moment after Ron told me that Mother and Dad will be moving to Texhoma Christian Care Center about six months from now. He said that Home Care is getting too expensive. I will have to go also if no one can be found to live with me in Dad's other house across the street from our home. (March 13)

Tonight, was entertaining for me at Akin Auditorium at MSU. There were parts of several operas performed by the MSU Opera Workshop. (March 15)

Mother had another flareup of her heart today. Debbie called 911 and an ambulance took Mother to ER at Bethania Hospital. The doctor said that Mother was having heart palpations. Steve took me to the "Y." (March 16)

Today I filled out the Sunday School record book. Attendance was down this week. (Sunday, March 17)

Jerry and Rita Allen came to the church for almost three hours looking at the By-Laws and Constitution. (March 18)

Sleet! Rain! Those were the two things that fell on Wichita Falls today. About 3:30 p.m. sleet began coming down hard. I had to ride my trike in it, but I managed to navigate home all right. I bought a new marimba today! (March 26) [The marimba was made by Yamaha.]

The original marimba was still useable. For a time, Shelby left his newer marimba at church and practiced on his older marimba at home. The mallets were replaced every two years, but the mallet holders only had to be replaced once and repaired several times in the fifty-three years that Shelby played his marimba.

I took off early today to get a feel of my new marimba by practicing several hours playing the songs that I will play at Monterey and the "Singspiration." Tonight, Clifford and I watched three chapters of a Tom Mix serial called "Miracle Rider" on his VCR. (March 28)

I spent the day at Hamilton Park watching tennis tournament matches. Tonight, I went to hear the Youth Symphony Orchestra at Akin Auditorium. (Saturday, March 30)

I went bowling today at Village Bowl and did okay. Scores in the two games were 100 and 134. Tonight, was the monthly "Singspiration." I played "Royal Telephone" and "In the Shadow of the Cross." (March 31)

I had to leave my job at 9:45 a.m. to go home and get my right shoe tied. While I was there, I got Mother to fix me some coffee. She was home by herself as Veronica took Dad to see about getting Medicaid. Tonight, Dan and I entertained the patients at Monterey Care Center playing eleven popular and country songs and three gospel songs. (April 2) [Veronica was employed as a fourth caretaker.]

Today I had to stay home with Mother and Dad because Debbie was sick and could not come. David came over with some homemade soup and stayed until Gladys came at 3:00 p.m. (April 6)

The HHBC choir put on an Easter program. Vivian and I did "The Old Rugged Cross Made the Difference" for the prelude. (April 7)

I am sick with the flu. I have a bad headache and have been coughing. I have been lying in bed, sitting in my recliner, and reading the newspaper all day. (April 8)

Another birthday with Shelby being sick. His sixtieth birthday was a far cry from his fiftieth when a large group of family and friends celebrated with him. He missed his second greatest joy in life, which came from being with large groups of family and friends. Playing his marimba to the glory of God was still his greatest joy. He ended his sixtieth year with a less positive attitude about his life. He liked his work and service at HHBC and enjoyed his many friends, but his family life was slimmer than ever, and he still had no female companion.

Mother's poor health prevented her from giving him the loving care that she had given him for fifty-nine years. Daddy was okay physically, but he showed increasing signs of senility. Ron lived 375 miles away in Jersey Village, Texas. Rod, Butch, and Jim lived 120 miles away in Fort Worth. David and Steve worked during the day and spent most of their evenings and nights with their families. But when his life darkened, Shelby always stood firm and did the best he could with what he had.

> Debbie told me that Ron called and said that he and Jeane would be here on Friday. Gladys took my temperature. It was 101 degrees. Aunt Lydia came over and gave me some Tylenol in liquid form. (Wednesday, April 10)
>
> Aunt Lydia came over to stay with Dad while Debbie took Mother to the doctor. Ron and Jeane came about 3 p.m. and stayed for six hours. (April 12)
>
> A three-hour meeting of the L. R. Stepp family was held this morning. Ron, David, Steve, Mother, Jeane, and I attended. Several things were discussed and decided. Two major ones were to move Mother and Dad to Texhoma Christian Care Center (TCCC) in about a month, and I would stay here. Working through an agency, efforts would be made to get Veronica and Lou Anne to help me. (April 13)

AN INCREDIBLE BOY AND A REMARKABLE MAN

> Having been sick for eight days, I got Debbie to take me to Wichita Falls Clinic. Dr. Frazier checked me over and diagnosed bronchitis. He gave me some antibiotics to take. (April 15)
>
> Today Ron turned 59. Unbelievable as it seems, he, Rod, and I are just a few years away from the rocking chair. At church, I was asked to serve on the Outreach Committee. I agreed to serve. (Wednesday, May 1)
>
> I worked all day hoeing weeds. (May 3)

Shelby's work at HHBC in 1996 was about two-thirds inside and one-third outside. He worked outside in both one hundred plus and almost freezing temperatures.

> Veronica took me to Dollar Saver to get two flashlights and some batteries. After supper, Gladys put the blue flashlight on the handlebar of my trike and the red one on the back of the basket for a taillight. (Saturday, May 4)
>
> Veronica took me to Park Place Living Center (PPLC) this morning. Mack Painter took us on a tour. Ron called me to ask what I thought about the place. I told him that I would give it a try for four or five days. (May 9)

On May 14, Shelby was introduced to the woman who would be his next-door neighbor at Park Place. Her name was Jeanette Averitt.

> I am in prison…errr, PPLC! Gladys brought me. I had to pay a whopping $640. I ate my first meal here. I had creamed potatoes, vegetable soup, potted meat, and milk shake. (Thursday, May 16)

The first full day of residency was shortened by seven hours of work at HHBC. Mack took me to and from work in his pickup. I sat out in the patio reading the newspaper. Nancy Adams who traded at Daddy's grocery store visited with me a while. (May 17)

The first full day at PPLC was spent eating breakfast, doing laundry, and sitting in the patio. My breakfast was oatmeal, scrambled eggs, and coffee. I was able to wash and dry my dirty clothes in the laundry room. In the patio I listened to the Preakness on my transistor radio and read the newspaper. (Saturday, May18)

After church I went with Aunt Lydia to see Mother and Dad at TCCC. This was their first day there. They both looked good and had a nice room. (Sunday, May 19)

I got stood up for an hour for my ride back to Park Place. Ike and Alma came to see me while I was eating supper. My advertisement in the newspaper seeking a Christian woman for companionship and possible mate ran for the first time today. (May 21)

I worked outside again today doing some more hoeing weeds. At 9:45 a.m., I took a break from work and went with Rusty Lynn to Taco Bell for a cup of coffee. Rusty had come to the church to water the flower beds. Mack picked up some chili, small cakes, and baby food for me. (May 22)

On this date, Ron had his third annual colonoscopy with polypectomy (not malignant) and again urged Shelby to have a colonoscopy.

I handed a note to Mack expressing my dissatisfaction with Park Place. Some reasons were:

trouble getting someone to tie my shoes, getting bath towels and rags in the bathroom, putting the bathroom mirror up, etc. Mack called David who had no solution. I gave Mack the phone number to call Ron, but he was too busy to call him. I had a good supper of chicken & dumplings, carrots, and vanilla pudding. (May 24)

David came up about 10 a.m. to take me to TCCC. Mother and Dad were looking good. Dad was on good behavior, not fussing to go home. David took me to my former home to get some more clothes. (Saturday, May 25)

Uncle Louis came back to do the bookkeeping at church. He had back surgery one month ago. He is helping Ken Davis get more acquainted with the book-keeping job he is about to take over from Louis who is resigning. I received two letters in response to my newspaper ad. One was from a lady in Electra and the other from a woman in Wichita Falls. Not sure about writing to the woman in Wichita Falls. (May 28)

The following from Rita Allen relates what Shelby did in response to "a woman in Wichita Falls."

Shelby put an ad in the classified section of our local newspaper. He was interested in meeting a single Christian lady. He got a response from a woman who was incarcerated, supposedly the first time, and she wanted to meet him. He asked me if I would take him. Against my better judgement, we went. When we got inside the jail they asked if he was on her visiting list, and he said that he was not. Then he was told that she was a regular who had been in jail numerous times. Shelby was disappointed. But he agreed not to pursue the meeting.

This evening while I was out in the courtyard at PPLC reading the paper, Jerry Allen and Ralph Piper surprised me with a Zenith portable TV. (Tuesday, June 4)

I got to go spend several hours visiting with Mother and Dad at TCCC. David took me and brought me home. (Saturday, June 8)

After breakfast I went over to Harold Jones Park [a few blocks away] for about three hours and read the paper while listening to bluegrass music. In the afternoon I went with Aunt Lydia to see Mother and Dad. We had another good visit with them. (Saturday, June 15)

For the third Sunday in a row, David had to provide my transportation to and from church. Before going there, David took me by my old home to get my other pair of shoes. I attended a Music Committee meeting at 5 p.m. (June 30)

The short work week was begun over on the parking lot hoeing weeds. I only got to do half of it. Veron Seay[3] a member of our church who had lent her TV to me while mine was being repaired, could not stand for me doing the work out in the hot sun so she did the rest. [She was age sixty-nine. He was age sixty.] I had a surprise visit by Uncle Ike and Alma around 6 p.m. (July 1)

Aunt Lydia bought me two pairs of Levi's and gave them to me when she took me to see Mother and Dad. Like other times, she took more goodies including bananas, watermelon, salmon, and Oreo cookies. I ate three cookies and drank a Pepsicola. (July 3)

> Today we celebrated the 120th birthday of our nation. I had my own picnic at Harold Jones Park. I had jars of Gerber's apricots, applesauce, a plastic container of Twinkies mixed with banana yogurt, and some Pepsi in a thermos. (July 4)
>
> Don [Erwin] took me and Ruth to church this morning. Ruth's car was out of service again, this time caused by a defective alternator. This afternoon Lydia and I went to see Mother and Dad. (Sunday, July 7)

Shelby took coffee breaks midmorning nearly every workday. His favorite place to go drink coffee was Taco Bell. Most of the time he rode his trike over there, but he often called someone to take him there and drink coffee with him. Ralph Piper joined him more than anyone.

> No YMCA today. I spent most of the morning out in the courtyard reading the Newsweek magazine and drinking coffee. Following a good lunch of steak with gravy, English peas, rice, and pound cake, I went over to Harold Jones Park to read and listen to my radio. Tonight, I took a can of tomato soup, a jar of Hawaiian Delight, and two cupcakes to the Church Cookout. (Saturday, July 13)
>
> The fifth Stepp-Bond reunion was held today in the Log Cabin at Lucy Park on the Wichita River. It was great to see my cousins. They included Charles Ray, Paul, and Lesley from the Bond clan; Mona and Norma of the Watkins; Butch and Rod from the Stepps, and Bob Vernon. Louis and Lydia and Mother and Dad were there. There were lots of good food. Desserts were homemade ice cream, lemon pie,

and German chocolate cake. I had some pie and ice cream. (July 20)

In Fellowship Hall a window was stuck, and I slammed my stubs against the pane to try to knock it loose. Doing so, I broke the glass and my right hand went through it. Fortunately, I escaped serious injury with only part of the skin scraped off. It bled profusely for a while. I kept dabbing it with a wet rag and the bleeding finally stopped. Aunt Lydia came to take me to TCCA. After we got there, she put some medication and a band-aid on it. We visited with Mother and Dad for a couple of hours, and then the four of us went to the cafeteria and ate some Strawberry-Blueberry pie. (July 26)

With my feet bothering me so much today, I could hardly get things done. (July 29)

I had a struggle all day in doing my work in the Sanctuary. I managed to finish endusting the pews and other furniture and sweeping and mopping the floor. My feet were hurting so bad that I couldn't run the vacuum on the rug. Nobody from PPLC ever came to pick me up. I called Ralph Piper who came and took me home. I had written him a $20 check while waiting, but when I offered it to him, he would not take it. (August 2)

While Aunt Lydia and I were visiting with Mother and Dad, Ol Shoemaker called and told me that my new shoes were ready. (August 3)

This morning Mack took me to the Little Ol' Shoemaker to get my new shoes. These are different from all the other shoes of mine. They have Velcro on the straps that I can fasten and unfasten. They include holes for shoestrings in case the Velcro quits working. (August 5)

AN INCREDIBLE BOY AND A REMARKABLE MAN

On August 6, 1994, second cousin once removed John B. "J. B." Ewing died at the age of eighty-four.

> Mother Nature teased the thirsty city of Wichita Falls today sending rain that fell heavy for a few minutes. Then just as fast as it started, it stopped just as quickly. Vivian and I brought the special music at church tonight. (Wednesday, August 7)
>
> When I arrived at work this morning, Uncle Ike and Aunt Alma were waiting for me in their car. The couple brought me some sausage and gravy, scrambled eggs, ground up bacon, and cantaloupe. After work I took it home with me. (August 9) Uncle Ike brought similar food to Shelby almost every Friday for several years.
>
> Ralph Piper took me to get an ice box [small refrigerator] at Walmart. I got in an electric cart and Ralph steered it. I found a General Electric one that I liked, so I bought it. (Thursday, August 22)
>
> Uncle Ike brought some more gravy with sausages, scrambled eggs, and a peach. He showed me how to use the microwave in the church kitchen. At dinner (lunch) time, I set the microwave at 30 seconds to heat the sausage and gravy to have with some tomato soup. (August 23)
>
> I phoned Mother this evening and she said she was taking oxygen because of breathing problems. (August 28)
>
> I received a phone call from Aunt Lydia telling me that Mother had been put in the hospital for a few days. (August 29)
>
> David and I went to the Bethania Hospital to see Mother this morning. Mother said that she was breathing better and sleeping better. Leaving

the hospital, David and I met Scroochie. He was going up to see Punkie who was seriously ill with congestive heart failure, one failed kidney and one barely functioning. (August 31)

On September 1, Ken Davis, church treasurer, began taking Shelby to church and back most Sunday mornings.

> I called Mother today and she said she was doing fine. (Tuesday, September 3)
> I received a letter from Ron today. He was happy to hear that I was making good adjustments at PPLC. He is going to do research and evaluate alternatives for me other than PPLC. Also, he planned on looking at redesigning my shoes. (September 4)
> I worked mostly in pain today, caused by either my calloused feet or shoes or both. It made me feel bad all over, thus I could not do a whole lot. I was reading the paper and listening to the radio when a Billy Graham Crusade series came on. Judy Garrison, a new resident came to sit down and talk for a few minutes. (September 5)
> David and I went out to see Mother. She was ill with her stomach. She has temporarily been placed in a room separate from Dad to get therapy and rest. David took me to Harold Park where I stayed for three hours. I ate a snack of two baby foods, an August apple fried pie, and some coffee. (Saturday, September 7)
> After church I sat out in the courtyard and read the paper. Judy and Jeanette came and sat at the table and visited with me. (September 8)
> While sitting in the dining room at PPLC eating supper, there was a tap on my right shoulder. I turned to look and there stood Ron and

Jeane. After visiting a little while in my room, the three of us went to see Mother at TCCC. She was doing better. She was sitting up in a chair and had just finished supper. Most of the conversation was about the times that Ronnie played baseball for the Panthers, Greyhounds, Broncos, and Riggers. (September 9)

Ron and Jeane stopped by to say goodbye this morning. Ron said he was going to call First Baptist Church Wichita Falls to see if they have a few members who could take me to events like Notre Dame High football games, Symphonies, basketball games, etc. (September 10)

This evening I attended a luncheon and missions program held by the WMU in Fellowship Hall. The emphasis of the program was on mission work in Texas. A puppet stage was set up like a TV news program. Rita Allen was the news anchor and the reporters were Jerry Allen, Stacey Clark, Frank Smith, and Al Claycamp. (Wednesday, September 11)

A part of me departed this earth this morning at 7:30. My dearest Mother left us with what appeared to be a fatal heart attack while sitting in a chair eating some oatmeal. David and Steve came at 9:15 to tell me. (September 12)

I went to work today since there was nothing for me to do in preparation for Mother's funeral. David was taking care of that. After dinner (lunch) I went over to Ray's Barbershop to get a haircut. This evening Ron and Jeane picked me up and we went to Hampton Vaughn's Funeral Home for the visitation and viewing Mother's body. She looked pretty dressed in a white blouse and black skirt. (September 13)

Mother's funeral was held today. Former HHBC Pastor Vernon Lewis did a splendid job. Rod, Butch, Jim, Steve, Don and Terry Erwin were the pallbearers. I was able to see a lot of cousins, aunts, and the two living uncles. On the Stepp side was Louis Watkins and on the Ewing side was Ike. David had family at his home for a meal afterwards. Ron and I learned that one of the hostess's was a daughter of Pat McNair, former second baseman of the Spudders. (September 14)

Mother was buried next to Daddy.

Ron and Jeane brought me some packages of underwear and four slipover shirts. He told me that I would have to go immediately and open a bank account in place of the joint account I had with Mother. They took me over to Norwest Bank where I opened a checking account. (Monday, September 16)

At work this morning I filled out the annual Sunday School report to go with the annual Church Letter. Rita Allen came in the office to review the recent S.S. literature that she had ordered. This evening out in the courtyard I visited with Judy and Jeanette. (September 17) [Shelby was "courting in the courtyard!]

Rita came to the church to check on some S.S. literature that was supposed to come in. At my request she made some new sheets for the record books for Sunday School. (Wednesday, October 9)

I rode my trike to Ray's to "get my ears lowered," but he was not there. So, I got my first haircut from a woman and she did a great job. The young lady barber is Linda. I left the barber shop and went to Radio Shack to get a new transistor radio which also aired the audio of TV channels like my old one. They did not have one, but they said they would get one tomorrow. (October 10)

This afternoon I practiced on some songs I planned to play for offertory and special music in the revival service tonight. My plan was wiped out because my foot was hurting me badly. (Monday, October 21)

The third revival service was held tonight. Roger Deerinwater preached on a Christian's reputation. I played "The King Is Coming." (October 22)

Tonight's revival service was another good one. Roger Deerinwater preached on the Christian's lack of interest in the lost people. His Bible text was Luke 10:13. Again I played a marimba solo. The song was "Canaanland Is Just in Sight." (October 23)

Jerry Allen provided my ride to prayer meeting tonight. Beginning tonight one of the deacons will do the same each Wednesday. (October 30) [Unfortunately, some of the deacons did not honor this commitment.]

This afternoon I was headed to my office when I saw Jeane coming up on the porch. I let her inside and she said that Ron was looking for me around the front. When he came where Jeane and I were, he said they had been at the old Stepp place getting Mother's and Dad's possessions placed in the center of each room for dividing up among the four brothers. (November 4)

This morning Ron and Jeane came and took me to Norwest Bank to get a safe deposit box. Ron had found my birth certificate and a $25 savings bond. I put both in the box. The bond and a $2 bill were given to me by Uncle Sonny in 1968. Ron was told that the savings bond would be worth $125 when it matures in 1998. (November 5)

I had a premonition that no one would call or come by and take me to the midweek service. Sure enough, that is exactly what happened. So, I spent a couple of hours reading the paper. (Wednesday, November 6)

Ron, David, Steve, and I got together at 3111 Avenue Q to decide who gets what of Mother's and Dad's possessions. Ron and Jeane had boxes of items in the middle of each room filled with stuff accumulated over 60 years. I took home a plaque, some books, and a footstool I had helped assemble at the Opportunity Workshop in 1965. (November 7)

The four Stepp brothers decided to sell their dad's home at 3111 Avenue Q.

In the morning worship service, Aunt Almeda and daughter Cynthia were guests of Aunt Ruth. Cynthia took me home in her new car. I thought somebody would call or come by and take me to church tonight, but nobody did. (Sunday November 10)

After work David took me to get the rest of my stuff out of the house. When I cleaned out my chest of drawers, I found an envelope with two $5 bills and a second envelope with a $20 bill. (November 11)

This was the Wednesday night for business meeting at church, but no one picked me up. (November 13)

Uncle Psychey Ikey brought me food tonight. He told me that Aunt Alma is having to go for some exams for 26 weeks to find out if she has Alzheimer's Disease. (Friday, November 15)

On this date exactly 33 years ago, President Kennedy was gunned down in Dallas while riding with John Connally in a motorcade. I was at Larry White's house watching a TV game show with him when the news bulletin flashed on the screen. (Friday, November 22)

At the "Y" today while reading the Times Record News, I saw a Kmart advertisement from which I picked out some novelty sports T-shirts for boys and girls that I thought about getting for Brandon and Brittany for Christmas. (November 23)

After two days of sleet, snow, and ice, the streets had just about been cleared and I was able to go to work. Tonight, David took me Christmas shopping. He would not let me get out and go into the stores because he knew the trouble that I was having with my feet. We went to Target and Walgreens. At both places I sat in David's truck and listened to some old rock & roll songs on his radio. (November 26)

At my request through a phone call, Ralph Piper came to take me to prayer meeting with him and Mary. The service was all prayer and testimonies. (Wednesday, November 27)

I had no place to go for Thanksgiving. David and Virginia had plans to visit her relatives. I had an accident this afternoon when I got back from the park. As I set foot on the newly waxed floor at the elevator, down I went. I hit my head on the edge of the right door frame and cut a gash over my right eye. I was taken to the

ER at Wichita General Hospital two blocks from here. They gave me a tetanus shot, cleaned and medicated the wound and put a band-aid on it. (November 28)

Well, on this date 55 years ago was one of the darkest hours in our nation's history. Pearl Harbor was surprisingly attacked by the Japanese. America lost 2,330 military personnel and civilians, 165 ships, and 1300 planes. (Saturday, December 7)

I started the big cleaning of endusting furniture, cleaning tables, chairs, lavatories, commodes, etc. in the Education Building. Then I vacuumed the rugs, swept and mopped the floors. (December 9)

I got a ride to church with Ralph Piper this evening. It was business meeting time with Jerry Allen presiding. (December 11)

This afternoon I started practicing some Christmas music on my marimba that I will play in the living room here on Saturday night. A Christmas Party is being held for the residents. In their personal cars, the PPLC staff took the residents to see the "The Fantasy of Lights" tonight. (Wednesday, December 18)

In addition to the cleaning duties I watered the poinsettias sitting on the platform and railings. I practiced for several hours on Christmas songs. (December 19)

I had a lot of visitors at work today. Uncle Ike started it with his weekly visit and bringing food for me. About 30 minutes later, Aunt Lydia came with some strawberry cake, chocolate cake, and cheese crackers. She also brought me some Christmas gifts. They were a sweater and black and white toboggan hat. Jack Stephens came to practice for two hours on Christmas songs we are going to play at the PPLC Christmas Party. (Friday, December 20) [This was Daddy's ninetieth birthday.]

The Christmas Party for the PPLC residents was held tonight with good attendance. I brought the music program playing both popular and sacred Christmas songs.

In the morning worship service, I played the special music. The song selected was "Away in A Manger." The church choir did a splendid job presenting a Christmas program of traditional Christmas hymns in the evening service. (December 22)

This is Christmas Eve and I have been sort of blue because of thinking about not having Mother around for the first in 60 Christmases. (December 24)

David came to get me at 9:30 this morning to take me to his house. We first went to TCCC to see Dad and take some gifts to him. Each of us gave him a shirt. From TCCC we went to see Steve and Debbie and give them and their girls some gifts. When we got to David's house, he and Virginia presented to me some gifts. They were a corduroy coat with a hood and a book titled Baseball's Greatest Games. Then we watched some "Amos and Andy Shows" on his VCR. (December 25)

Tonight, was our monthly Singspiration. It was another good one. Jerry Allen's brother J. D. "Sammy" did a song by himself, one song with his son, and one song with Jerry's daughter Cheryl and Cheryl's son. I played "Then I Met the Master" and "Royal Telephone." (December 29)

Well, it is hard to believe that we are in the final hours of 1996. With two hours left, I am sitting at a table in the smoking room reading the paper and looking at a New Year's Eve Special on TV. With me are Jeanette Averitt, Gary Carpenter, Henry, D. J. Collins, and Charlie. (Tuesday, December 31)

In 1997, Shelby retired from work at HHBC. His callouses on both leg stubs were causing pain when he was on his "feet" a lot of the time while working. Back in the 1970s, he had surgery to remove similar callouses, but the pain during the surgery and recovery caused him to never consider doing that again.

His schedule of daily activities for the rest of 1997 and all of 1998 were similar to 1996 except without employment and with courting Jeanette. David, Uncle Ike, Aunt Lydia, and Jerry and Rita Allen continued to visit him, provide transportation, etc. When Ron and Jeane visited Daddy in the Alzheimer unit at TCCC in 1997, Daddy called Ron, "Hoss." When Daddy and Uncle John were teenagers on their dad's farm near Hugo, John called Lee Roy "Monk" and Lee Roy called John "Hoss." So, now and in the future, Ron acted like he was "Hoss" and Daddy was "Monk." Neither Ron nor Jeane thought that Daddy had Alzheimer's disease because he was more cognizant than the other residents in that unit. In May of 1998, Ron and Jeane visited Daddy, and it was obvious that he did not recognize Ron as his son nor as "Hoss" but just someone that he knew. He did still recognize Shelby, David, and Aunt Lydia.

On June 2, 1998, Jerry and Rita took Shelby to a Texas Ranger game in Arlington, Texas, as mentioned by Rita on page 204.

About the same time, Ron and Jeane's house on Lake Livingston was completed. However, they could not move there because Jeane's mother who lived with them in Jersey Village would not agree to live there. She wanted to continue living next door to Ron Alan, Debbie, Brandon, and Brittany. Ron had already resigned at St. Christopher Episcopal Church, but he soon was hired by Jersey Village Baptist Church as minister of administration with a salary almost double his recent salary.

David called Ron on January 6, 1999, and told him that Daddy had just died. He was ninety-four years old. His life span was longer than any Stepp that they knew. The theme of Lee Roy's funeral service was repeated numerous times by former HHBC pastor, Max Dowling. It was "He was a good man, he was an honest man, and he was a hardworking man." Daddy was buried next to Mother.

A few days after Daddy's funeral, Shelby called Ron and asked for his permission to marry Jeanette. Of course, Shelby was free to do as he wished in this matter, but because Ron had taken care of all the official and legal requirements in place of Mother, Dad, and Shelby since 1994, he wanted Ron's okay. Ron told Shelby that he was happy to support him in this big decision.

On Valentine's Day of 1999, Shelby and Jeanette were married at HHBC. Jerry Allen was Shelby's best man. Robert Brazile conducted the marriage ceremony. Soloist Gail Piper, one of Ralph's daughters, sang "Always." A reception followed in Fellowship Hall. Attendance was good at both events. Shelby finally had his long-awaited female companion.

Nine months later, Shelby and Jeanette moved to Alterra Sterling House where they had good accommodations, service, activities, and meals. In their first year, they enjoyed each other, buying furniture—something Shelby had never done—and making new friends.

In 2000 and 2001, Shelby's daily routine included reading the newspaper, listening to his transistor radio, and enjoying time with his wife and several other friends at Alterra. He practiced his marimba every day with a few exceptions and played at church three or four times each month. He played his compact discs of classical, country, and other music weekly. Occasionally, he played his marimba for some of the residents at Alterra. He rode his trike for about thirty minutes in the parking lot when weather permitted.

Beginning in February 2002, Shelby started entertaining the Alterra residents twice each week on Monday and Thursday. He played marimba solos and accompanied the attendees while they sang hymns, popular and other songs. He selected the songs and enlisted the emcee and soloists.

Following are selected entries from Shelby's diary of 2002.

I got a call and was told that my mallet cuff was ready. I had nobody available to pick it up until Friday. Tonight, there were more people than usual at my marimba musical—he soon would call it, "An Evening in Marimba Land." There was a new lady who had just moved in yesterday. She came to Jeanette and me after the program and introduced herself as Lynn Foster. She expressed how much she enjoyed my music. I was surprised to learn that she and her family are good friends with Aunt Nila and Cousin Jim Ewing. (Thursday, February 14) [This was his third wedding anniversary. Surely, Shelby did not forget that.]

I got my repaired mallet cuff back today. It works fine. The man who did the welding did not charge me anything. I rode my trike around in the parking lot for about thirty minutes even though it was very windy. (February 15)

It sure was pleasant today. I rode my trike again and enjoyed it more than yesterday. Tonight's "Chicken Foot" winner—"Toot Toot"! She is either close to my number of wins or may have surpassed mine. (February 16)

"Chicken Foot" is a domino game that Shelby, Jeanette, and four or five others played almost daily. Shelby won the most games, and Jeanette won the next most games. Shelby began calling Jeanette "Toot Toot" early after their marriage, but that was his personal and private nickname for her. So, she will be referred to as Jeanette from this point forward including replacing it in his diary entries.

Jeanette got up at 6:30 a.m. and took some more clothes to the laundry room. It was too early for me so I stayed in bed until 7:30. When she got back she did some dusting. I was hoping that her doing chores would make her feel better about herself and get on the road to recovery from depression.

This afternoon, Uncle Ike took us to Maplewood Eye Center to get new frames for Jeanette's two lenses and to put one of my lenses back in the frames. Then he took us to Wells Fargo to do some banking, and he took us to Hester's Hearing Aids to repair one of her hearing aids. When we got back to Alterra, Uncle Ike put some tire sealer in my trike tires and aired them up. (Tuesday, February 19)

I practiced for about two hours and then Jeanette and I relaxed on the front porch. It was such a beautiful day, I got my trike out on the parking lot after lunch and rode around for about 30 minutes. (February 20)

About 11:00 a.m. Glenn told Jeanette that she would be going to Red River Hospital (RRH) after lunch. This really upset her. Glenn explained to her that she needed to go there so she could get her medication regulated. We went to RRH and were told that she would be undergoing tests and evaluations. I never got to talk to Dr. Bibb who was her doctor. I went back to Alterra and conducted the Thursday night music program. The program went smoothly. Afterwards I had some extra help from Lynn Foster who picked up the hymnals and put them away. As I sit here in my room, the feeling of loneliness is already overshadowing me. (February 21)

I had trouble contacting Jeanette by phone. Finally, Jerri at RRH said that she would get Jeanette and call me. When the call came, I picked up the receiver and said "hello." She answered.

> I asked how she was doing, and she said "fine." Later I told her that I would be coming to see her at 5 p.m. I then told her I loved her. She replied that she loved me too. (Friday, February 22)
>
> I had a little better luck talking to Jeanette this afternoon than I did this morning. She seemed to be more alert. I asked her how her day was going and she said she stayed in her room all day and slept the biggest part of the time. I told her to stay out of the room as much as she could because she wasn't helping herself doing that. She said that nobody would talk to her. I came right back and told her that sometimes you have to speak first to open a conversation. (February 23) [Shelby would soon learn that "sometimes you have to speak not."]

For four years, Red Winn and wife, Linda, provided transportation for Shelby and Jeanette regularly to Sunday school and morning church services. Linda did some of their laundry service and other needs. Their Sunday school teacher, Travis Street, also provided transportation to the Wednesday night service.

> We had another good marimba concert and a great job done by Frances in emceeing for me. I had some additional help from Jimmy Stewart and Lynn Foster. Jimmy passed out the hymnals and Lynn put the sheet music on my music stand for me. (February 26)
>
> This morning when I got up from the table, the bottom of my left foot started hurting as soon as the shoe touched the floor. I was able to walk down the hallway for a short distance, but then I had to get down on my knees and walk on them the rest of the way to my apartment. After I lied

down for a while, I got up to see if I could walk without pain. I could. (Friday, March 1)

After twelve days at RRH, Jeanette came back to Alterra.

Someone from RRH brought Jeanette back home around 5:30 p.m. I was eating at the time. After supper I went to the apartment and was so glad to see her. We hugged, kissed, and I told her it was a relief to have her back. I went to get someone to hang up Jeanette's laundered clothes, but no workers were available. As I went back to the apartment, Lynn Foster was fixing to unlock her door. I asked if she would take care of Jeanette's clothes. She so kindly agreed and did a good job. (March 4)

While Hank was giving me a haircut, I brought up the subject of baseball and that the major league season was only three weeks away. I mentioned that the Texas Rangers should do better with their addition of Chan Ho Park. Hank said that with so many teams there are no longer superstars like Willie Mays, Mickey Mantle, Joe Dimaggio, Ralph Kiner, and Hank Greenberg. I certainly agreed with him. (March 6) [Two Yankees, one Giant, one Pirate, one Detroit Tiger, and no Dodger, and Shelby agreed with him. Even worse, he wrote it in his diary.]

In the mail today came a letter and brochure from Jamall Badry. [He was a longtime music evangelist and the executive director of the Colorado Springs-based Music Evangelism Foundation.] He asked if I could come help him by playing on a Monday night, June 24th in Colorado Springs in the first night of the Annual

Bible Conference. I told Jeanette that I hoped to find someone to take me this year. (March 7)

I called Ron and asked how Brandon was doing. Ron said Brandon was walking now and throwing a baseball. The surgeon said that we should know in a month whether Brandon might play baseball again. (Saturday, March 9)

Brandon had major surgery on his right leg after an accident at a Whataburger. It happened after a baseball game when he got up to leave. The floor had been mopped while he was eating. He was wearing his kid baseball rubber cleats, and his feet when out from under him, and he landed on his right knee. He was taken to an ER. The following day, he had surgery that took four and a half hours to reattach a ligament. They had to drill a hole in his tibia just below the knee, pull the end of the ligament through the hole, and fasten it to a metal button. It appeared that his football and baseball days were over.

I went with Red Winn to the Brotherhood breakfast this morning at Trinity Baptist Church. Red used the blender to prepare the eggs so I could eat them. One of the items brought up by Red in the short business meeting was to present to the church a motion to pay for some new mallets and mallet cuffs for me. (March 10)

We had another good crowd at Monday night's "An Evening in Marimba Land." After the program Joy Steward visited with us in our apartment. She presented the plan of salvation to Jeanette, and within forty minutes she was converted. We got down on our knees and Jeanette repeated after Joy the sinner's prayer. (March 11)

I had called David and asked for $200 to be used to purchase some much needed clothes and other necessities. This evening he brought a check made out to me for the full amount. (March 14)

Jeanette got her hair fixed this afternoon and saved ten dollars. Lynn Foster did her hair and did a fine job. Jeanette invited her to our apartment to have some Dr Pepper. I drank some coffee. Then Bonnie Hill took us shopping to get some new clothes. After shopping Bonnie and Jeanette decided to stop at Scott's Hamburger Drive-In and got some burgers. (March 15)

We had Uncle Ike over to eat dinner with us shortly after noon. He had an unfavorable report on Aunt Ruby. He went with Aunt Almeda and Cousin Nelson to the nursing home in Weatherford. They found the poor lady suffering with Alzheimer's and respiratory problems. It is amazing to me that the 85-year-old precious woman has come this far. (Saturday, March 16)

Psychie Ikie brought me some more Chow Chow. It was better than all he had brought before. He said that he added some green onion this time. It was sure delicious on top of the meat dish I ate. We talked and watched a Pete Sampras—Lleyton Hewitt tennis match. Psychie Ikie will be going on a 2400-mile trip. He will spend the first night with Barbara and Jerry Rogers in Starkville, Mississippi. From there he will go to Atlanta, Georgia, to visit his daughter Pam and her husband. Then he will be on to Detroit, Michigan, to see Phillip. On the way back home, he will stop at a small town in West Texas to see Imogene's granddaughter. (March 17)

On the day every year, Aunt Laverne and my schoolteacher Thelma Thompson celebrated their birthday. Both are deceased. The former would be 96 and the latter 102. (March 18)

This evening at Trinity Baptist Church, I played at the beginning of the wedding of Forrest Cotton and Maggie Jackson. The song was "Love Me Tender" and my accompanist was Merle Hoeffner. (March 24)

There was a good gathering for "An Evening in Marimba Land." Jeanette told the audience that I may get an all expenses paid trip to Colorado Springs to play, for the third time, in the Music Evangelism Foundation's Annual Bible Seminar. Everyone was impressed and gave me a big applause. I nodded my head in appreciation to them. (March 25) [The remainder of his diary for 2002 is missing.]

Shelby celebrated his sixty-sixth birthday on April 8.

A couple from Trinity Baptist Church, Tom and Jo Ann Malaise, graciously took Shelby to Colorado Springs, Colorado. Jo Ann was the pianist at Trinity Baptist Church. On June 25, 2002, at Village Seven Presbyterian in Colorado Springs, Colorado, Shelby played his marimba at their annual Music Evangelism Foundation Bible Seminar. After playing his marimba, Shelby received a standing ovation from the audience of about 2,500. This was the third and last time that Shelby was able to accept their invitation. Shelby said in the last year of his life that he enjoyed and got more fulfillment in playing at those three events than any in his life. Ron wishes today that he and Mother could have been there for at least one of them. A photo of Shelby playing there is included in this book.

On September 24, 2002, Aunt Ruby Ewing Stepp Faulkenberry died in Weatherford, Texas, at the age of eighty-six. Ron presented her eulogy. Shelby and Ron had lost their "second Mother."

Uncle Louis M. Watkins died on October 8, 2002, at the age of eighty-two.

Teddie Loreda Bills Curfman, Jeane's mother, died on November 6, 2002, at the age of eighty-seven in Houston, Texas. She was "Granny" to Ron's family after Brandon and Brittany were born.

AN INCREDIBLE BOY AND A REMARKABLE MAN

Ron presented the eulogy, which included, "She was the best mother-in-law one could have. She never said a negative word to me." She was buried next to Webb. She is often remembered in conversations of Ron, Jeane, Ron Alan, Brandon, and Brittany.

Selected entries from Shelby's diary of 2003 follow:

> We had company for a couple of hours this morning and part of the afternoon as Uncle Psychie Ikie came to see us. I had called him and after he agreed to come, I had made arrangements and paid the $6 to reserve the Sunroom. He had another sack of goodies for us. He brought a jar of beets for Jeanette and a jar of his homemade Chow Chow for me. (Monday, June 10)
>
> At 4:30 p.m. I received a phone call from Ron. He was calling from the Hampton Inn where he and Jeane usually lodge when they come to Wichita Falls. He said that they were beginning a one-week vacation trip. He asked if we had any plans tonight. I told them we were as usual going to play Chicken Foot. Ron asked if I wanted them to come afterwards, I told him to come on at 6:30, we can miss Chicken Foot tonight.
>
> We all sat in the Sunroom and had a good two-hour visit. Ron said that Brandon is doing well with the therapy treatments for his leg. Another thing that I learned is that Ron Alan and his wife had bought a 3-acre property for $90,000 and are having a house built on it.
>
> We started talking about the all-time famous movie stars. I said that Robert Taylor was my favorite actor and Susan Hayward was my favorite actress. Ron said that he liked Gary Cooper, John Wayne, Spencer Tracy, and Gregory Peck (who incidentally died yesterday). His favorite

actress was Maureen O'Hara. I asked them to join us at Trinity Baptist Church tomorrow and eat dinner with us at Alterra. They consented. (Saturday, June 4)

Today is the day we honor our fathers, living and deceased. This is the fifth year that I, Ron, David, and Steve will be without our dad. At our worship service, I introduced Ron and Jeane to many of our church members. Following the luncheon in the Sunroom at Alterra, we went out to the graves of Mother and Daddy. I sat down by their graves thinking in almost unbelief that Mother has been gone six years and Dad four and a half years. I thought of how well they took care of me and the 60 years I lived with them. Ron and Jeane had gone to another area of the cemetery where their first son was buried.

Then we drove to Riverside Cemetery where our Grandparents Stepp are buried. We had to walk up an incline about thirty yards to the graves. Ron helped me and Jeane helped Jeanette, but she did not make it all the way. We rode around for about 40 minutes after leaving Riverside, and then Ron took us home. (June 15)

Ralph Piper, as always was right on time to pick me up and take us to Braum's for coffee. We shared what each had been doing since we last visited together. (Tuesday, June 24)

After riding my trike, I was back to my marimba to practice for tonight's songs. My arms shook badly and it was a struggle getting through all 14 songs. I decided to try using one mallet with both stubs and no cuffs. At the program this evening I played the first four songs with the single mallet and found out that did not work. My arms got so sweaty I could not hold the mallet well. I got Jeanette to go get my cuffs with mallets. I was able to play all the program without shaking. (June 30)

Dixie from Health Pro Home Health Services took me to Sam Gibbs Music to buy a pair of mallets. They cost $30. She insisted on paying for my two new mallets. When I resisted, she told me to please let her so she could feel good about helping me. I finally consented and thanked her. (July 3)

We had a special dinner at Alterra on this special day. We were served hot dogs, potato salad, baked beans, and cole slaw. The dessert was apple pie. I was disappointed when informed there would be no SAFB fireworks show. (July 4)

After several weeks of struggling while playing his marimba with only one mallet using both stubs with no cuffs, Shelby finally got his modified cuffs with his two new mallets.

Gaylon from Call Field Boots & Shoe Repair brought my cuffs with mallets attached. I put on the cuffs and tried them out on my marimba by playing "There's a Tear in My Beer" and they worked just fine. I was able to play the song to the end without any pain or shaking. I thanked Gaylon for his work. (Tuesday, July 15)

At church I was able to play the offertory and special music without any stiffening in my arms. I thanked God for putting His hands on my shoulders during that time. (Sunday, August 10)

I had a terrible time practicing again as my arms and shoulders acted up once more. During the program tonight, Psychie Ikie played three songs on his harmonica. They were "Precious

Memories," "Amazing Grace," and "Home On the Range." Ike was followed by a sing-along of "On Top of Old Smokey" and "Red River Valley." This program was one of the best I have had in a long time. (August 11)

I was able to play the entire program with cuffs and mallets with hardly any difficulty. (August 14)

I had a rough evening playing the marimba as my left arm and shoulder bothered me. I had to stop every few minutes to relax the muscles. With determination, I made it to the end. (Thursday, August 21)

David came to visit us tonight. We talked about the good times when there was real rock and roll music of the '50s and '60s, about stars like Elvis Presley, Ray Charles, Buddy Holly, Bo Diddly, Chuck Berry, Little Richard, Big Bopper, Ritchie Valens, etc. David said that Jim had bought some land near Nocona worth $100,000, and planned to build a house. We had a nice one-hour visit. (August 22)

I did something this morning that was quite an accomplishment for me. Despite a struggle, but with determination, I managed to unlock the lock on the part of the chain wrapped around the trike chain and panel. How I did it was to hold the lock between my legs, stick the key in the keyhole, turn the key to the right, and it unlocked. I did this because no Alterra employees were available to unlock it. (August 24)

Again, no one was available to unlock my bike, so I was fortunate to unlock it myself again. After riding my trike I went back to my apartment and decided to drink a can of grape juice. However, with Jeanette gone to the doctor, I had no one to open the can. I grabbed a little knife (paring knife), pushed the pointed end of it under the flap on the top of the can and raised it half-way up. I took hold of the flap with my stubs and pulled it open. (Tuesday, August 26)

I had some trouble trying to play with two mallets once more. I tried playing with the left mallet for two songs and then the right mallet for two songs, etc. I did okay with the left mallet, but when playing with the right mallet the muscles in my right arm tightened to where I could not move the mallet forward to hit a key. After the first two songs, I played the remaining songs with the left mallet. (Saturday, August 30)

When we got back home, I was delighted to have my favorite dish—hot dog [chili dog]. (Wednesday, September 3)

I was a one-handed/mallet marimba player in the worship service. I told Charles Medlin about the problems with my shoulders and arms. During the time members were meeting and greeting, Charles came to me and put his hands on my shoulders and said a prayer for me. I thanked him for doing so. (Sunday, September 14)

Uncle Ike came to visit us today. He said that he had just been to Clinics of North Texas to make an appointment tomorrow with his doctor to undergo a blood-thinning procedure. We had the sprite 82-year-old fellow with us for about three hours. We spent an hour of that time eating lunch here. (Wednesday, October 8)

The inevitable happened. My trike was stolen either last night or two nights ago. I discovered it missing when I went out after lunch to the spot behind a fence where it was always parked. I could not lock the bike as I usually do because the grass was still wet from the water sprinkler running the night before, and I did not want to get my pants wet. I could not call the police because Jeanette was gone to the doctor. Later, when she returned and I told her my trike was missing, she called the police and reported that.

A young policeman came ten minutes after the call. He got all the pertinent information about the trike including color, brand name, serial number, and size. Then he got my personal information. He said sometimes the thief takes the stolen item to a pawn shop. He stated there are five pawn shops around town and he and other policemen would be checking with them weekly to see if my trike can be located. In tonight's program I mentioned the missing trike and asked those attending to pray that it either be returned to me or that another trike be provided for me. (Monday, October 27)

I was taken in the Alterra [sometimes referred to as Sterling House or Alterra Sterling House] van to the Times-Record News to pay for the trike ad. The cost was $18.98, and I wrote out a check for that amount. (Wednesday, October 29)

Someone from TV Channel 3 called Jeanette and asked permission to come and interview Shelby about his stolen trike and take video to be aired tonight and or tomorrow. Soon after the call, Mikel Tellith, a TV3 reporter came out with a video recorder and other equipment. She asked what I usually did during the morning hours. Jeanette, speaking for me, told her that I usually practice on my marimba. Mikel asked that we go where it is so she could video record me playing.

AN INCREDIBLE BOY AND A REMARKABLE MAN

While Mikel was taking some recordings. I played a couple of songs that were on my program tonight. She then had me to walk away from the marimba and go around the corner like I was going back to the apartment. She then had me reverse and head back toward the marimba while she recorded that.

Then we went to the apartment and she had us sit down and carry on a conversation with each other while she recorded. Mikel then asked Jeanette, while the recording continued, what her reaction was when she heard my trike was stolen. She said she could not understand how anyone could get so low to do such a thing.

Mikel then wanted to get one of the other resident's reaction. It was dinner time, and we went to the dining room. Jeanette told Mikel that we had a good lady friend named Francis Burleson. When Francis was told what Mikel wanted from her for the recording, she looked at me with a smile and quipped, "Aha, this is my chance." She was kidding about having the opportunity to tell people how bad I was. Mikel asked Francis what her reaction was when she heard my trike was stolen. Francis said she was real upset about it and hoped whoever took it would have a change of heart and return it.

I asked Mikel what time the interviews would be on TV this evening. She said that they would be on at five and six o'clock. This evening at 5 p.m. we watched the first part of the newscast about my stolen trike. It showed me walking up the hallway part showing the front of Sterling House, me walking up the hallway toward my marimba, and Jeanette talking. At 6 p.m. the newscast showed me playing the marimba, Francis talking, and the front of Sterling House. A newscaster named Emily reported that a woman had called to offer her bike to me. (November 10)

This morning Glenn [Dickens, Sterling House resident director] told me that a woman had called and wanted to give her 3-wheeler to me. Earlier another lady called from Henrietta to say that she and her husband wanted to buy a new 3-wheeler for me. With the two offers, I was caught between a rock and a hard place, not knowing which of the offers to accept. I have always been leery of second-hand stuff. Since Glenn was kind enough to offer to take us to the lady who offered her used trike, we decided to go have a look at it.

When arriving at the address we were given, Glenn went to the first apartment and knocked on the door. Out came a short elderly lady with short grey hair. She identified herself as Lilian Ward and said that she knew me since I was a little kid, and that she traded at Dad's "little grocery store." She went to a fiberglass shed, unlocked the door, and there sat a royal blue 3-wheeler with the white spokes in the three wheels. Much to my surprise the trike was in real good condition. Lilian said that she had the trike for seven years, but only got to use it two of those years.

Since Lilian had known me and my parents a long time, I accepted her gift. While waiting for Sterling House Community Sales Representative Carolyn Spencer's husband to come and get the trike and haul it to Sterling House, Lilian talked to Glenn and me. She said my mother showed she had a mother's compassion for me as she always worried about my well-being. (Tuesday, November 11)

AN INCREDIBLE BOY AND A REMARKABLE MAN

Ron and Jeane came to see us this afternoon. They visited with us for about an hour and then went to Hampton Inn to check in, wash up, and change clothes. Upon our invitation, they came back to dine with us in the Sunroom. We had turkey and dressing provided by Sterling House and sweet potatoes, green beans, and other food brought by some of the resident's families.

After the dinner I provided the entertainment on my marimba playing three or four songs and ending with "God Bless America." With the latter song, I had the audience sing along while playing it a second time. Before I started playing, Ron stood by me and gave a brief bio of my life. And when I started playing, he told about the time I played at a WFSH Assembly in 1954. Ron said that he was surprised when the curtains opened and there was a marimba like mine on stage. He felt for sure that the marimba was mine and that I would be playing it. He told the people that I not only played it, but also did some tap dancing at the end.

After the program, Ron and I along with Jeanette and Jeane visited in the living room for about 90 minutes. I told Ron about my right arm still giving me some trouble. He mentioned that Kathleen Coker does massage therapy, and that he would call her tomorrow and see if she would come out and do therapy on my arms and shoulders. He asked if I would agree to such treatments, and I said that I would.

Ron asked if we had any plans for tomorrow morning. I answered that as of right now we do not. He said that they were going to Charlie to buy some pecans at Chitwood's Pecan Farm like they have done for many years, and that Mother had done for many years before that. He thought we would enjoy the ride. Jeanette and I were for doing that since we seldom have such opportunities to go places other than to the doctors. (Friday, November 21)

As we headed toward Charlie, Ron drove through parts of Wichita Falls to a few old familiar sights including Lee Street where Lloyd and Floyd Stone grew up, Fat Boys hamburger joint, and where Spudder Park used to be. At the Westside Farmers Ranch Foundation Pecan Shop, Ron bought $120 worth of pecans—Barton and Mohawk. They were $2 per pound.

Our next stop was at Sikes Senter Mall where I tried to find an 18" gold chain for Jeanette's silver and gold pendant that I got for her on our first wedding anniversary. She could not handle the walking so Ron took her back to the apartment. Back at the mall we went to Penny's jewelry department. Jeane put the pendant on an 18" silver and gold chain and tried it on. It was too short. She then tried a 20' chain that fit, but it did not have the same design as the old one. We had to walk a further distance to Zale's Jewelry, but did not have any luck there either.

I sat down in a rest area, while Ron and Jeane went to Gordon's Jewelry. About 20 minutes later they came back with what they thought for sure was the right chain. When Ron dropped me off at the apartment, I presented the little red box with the 20" gold chain and pendant inside. She first thought it was not the right size, but putting it around her neck she found it suited her.

Ron and Jeane came back to Sterling House later for Jeanette's birthday party. After the party, the couple spent two hours with me and Jeanette in our apartment before they were to head back to Houston tomorrow morning. Ron gave me a present I had been asking for. It was some cassette tapes of several old Lone Ranger radio shows from December of 1943 and February of 1944. We had probably heard them when they aired on those dates. Ron put on one of the tapes and we listened to a little bit of the first two stories. The Couple left at about 9 o'clock, and I reckon we won't see them again until next spring. (Saturday, November 22)

I played my marimba at the Royal Estates of Wichita Falls Senior Living Apartments for the second time. I played nine songs, closing out with a song appropriate for Thanksgiving season called "Let Us Break Bread Together." In the audience were two old friends from HHBC, Mary Lou Rigsby and Mrs. Sparks. Mary Lou's son was there from San Antonio to be with his mother for Thanksgiving. (Wednesday, November 26)

After extensive tests and exams, Dr. Pena arranged for me to have a physical therapist to start giving me physical and occupational therapy regularly at my apartment. He told me to see him again in three or four months. (Tuesday, December 16)

Just before the Choir presented the Christmas Cantata, I played my marimba during the offertory accompanied by Jo Ann Malaise. The song was "What Child Is This?." The choir did well in singing the cantata. It was followed by the observance of The Lord's Supper. (Sunday, December 21)

Aunt Sis and Andrew came for a visit this afternoon. We took them to the Sunroom for a short thirty-minute visit. Aunt Sis gave us the stunning news that Uncle Ike was diagnosed of having lung cancer. She said that they were going to have Christmas with Cynthia and her husband in Dallas. Cynthia was to come and pick them up tomorrow or Wednesday. Aunt Sis had another surprise for us, she gave each of us a fifty-dollar bill. We gave them hugs and expressed how grateful we were for them to give us the money. (December 22)

Jeanette and I did not open our gifts for each other until after dinner. She was real pleased with the red blouse and socks. I felt the same about the gold chain she gave me for my wedding ring. (December 25)

Santa Claus paid a day after Christmas visit to us in the person of David. This morning he brought me the clothes that I had asked for. They were two sets of pajamas, two slip-over shirts, two sweaters, three black dress jeans, two blue jeans, two dress shirts, and two ties. He brought Jeanette a tweed jacket. We were pleased with our gifts and expressed our thanks to David. Later, Jeanette's son, Don, came for a short visit and gave us a $200 check made out to Jeanette. (December 26)

Merri, Jeanette's daughter came to visit today and brought a big gift box for her. When she opened the box, she pulled out a pant suit and three blouses and said she was thrilled to get them. Merri told me that I am not left out because she is going to take me shopping tomorrow to get my gifts. Jeanette had a list of errands for tomorrow and one included going to the bank to deposit the $200 check from Ron and Jeane, and the same from Don. (December 28)

Today is the beginning of a new year. For the first year since I can't remember when, I did not watch the Rose Parade. I was more interested in sitting in the Sunroom and reading the newspaper. Also, I only watched the Orange Bowl and Rose Bowl. (Thursday, January 1, 2004)

I called Aunt Lydia this afternoon and had another nice visit. I told her that the rheumatologist said that he thought I had muscular arthritis. She said that she went to be with Mona, Jim, and their family for the Christmas holidays. She also stated that Mona will soon have surgery to repair a heart valve. She gave an update on Norma and Steve's family. Nathan is applying for a job with the National Oceanic Association, Seth is in college, and Ian is in his senior year at WFSH. (January 2)

Jeanette brought me a letter from Dr. Lucy Tan stating that I had sclerosis of the spine. This afternoon we went in the Alterra van to an appointment with Dr. Pena. He said that my sclerosis was caused by a lack of fluid, but also my spine was not straight. He had me take a bone scan. Following the procedure, I asked when the results would be reported. She said it would be about one week. Dr. Pena told me that the results of the blood tests were good and ruled out diabetes, lupus, rheumatoid arthritis, and my cholesterol level was good. He made me an appointment to see him on February 24th. (Tuesday, January 13)

Norman Wilde, a resident at Sterling House, had told me several times that he would like to sing "Tell It to Jesus." Saturday morning and afternoon and again this morning, I worked with him on that song. This evening I billed him as my "guest artist." Norman got a big applause for the good job of singing. Jeanette told him that he had a good baritone voice, and Francis agreed. (Monday, February 2)

This was a very special day for two reasons. One, it was our fifth wedding anniversary and we also attended the annual Sterling House Valentine's Day Party. We had snow falling from early morning to early afternoon. The five and a half inches was the most in WF in twenty years. (Saturday, February 14)

Ron called this evening and said they plan to come up in two weeks. I gave him an update on our health issues. (Saturday, February 21)

I kept an appointment this afternoon with Dr. Pena who told me that I would have to start medication to strengthen my bones. Since I cannot physically swallow the Actonel pill, I will have to get injections of Forteo daily for six months to a year. I was furious when he told me that. He said that he would give me the first one now, but I refused it. He gave me a brochure on Forteo and Osteoporosis. I'm going to have to do some tall thinking on whether to take Forteo injections. (February 24)

Ron and Jeane came to see us about 1:30 p.m. and visited for a few hours. We talked mostly about the Forteo injections. After reading the booklet on Osteoporosis and pamphlet on Forteo, Ron urged me to start getting the injections. I asked about Ron Alan and his wife, and Ron said they were doing fine are about finished with the construction of their "mansion." Ron said that 13-year-old Brandon was almost as

AN INCREDIBLE BOY AND A REMARKABLE MAN

tall as Ron Alan, and his rehab was coming along well enough for him to jog. (Saturday, February 28)

Ron and Jeane picked us up at 3 p.m. and said they had a long visit with Ruth Franklin at TCCC. Ruth is the mother of Howard who was one of Ron's teammates on the Greyhounds and Broncos. We went to see Uncle Ike and had a good visit under the circumstances of him dying of lung cancer and coughing a lot. Ron asked him about what he did in the Navy during WWII, his memories of childhood and places where he lived with his parents.

The lung cancer is taking its toll on Uncle Ike and he is looking frail. He has lost 40 pounds. My left shoe gave me fits again on the way back to Ron's car, and he and Jeane had to help me walk in the grass. (February 29)

Ron picked me up mid-morning and took me to the shoe shop. I told Gaylon how bad the shoe hurt and what I think needed to be adjusted. Gaylon said he would give it a try, but I would have to leave the shoe a few days. When we got back home Ron said they needed to hit the road and make the 375-mile trip back to Jersey Village. We all hugged, and they left. (March 1)

Brandon was able to play baseball again. He did not run as fast as before, but he fielded well at shortstop and hit well. But during spring break, his family went skiing at Breckenridge Resort in Colorado, and Brandon rented "trick skis" and went down a double black diamond slope[4] without his dad's permission. A woman who saw him "wipe out" said that he somersaulted six times and neither ski binding ever released. It took the rangers several hours to get him down the slope and to the ER. It was determined that he fractured both tibias and fibulas. Surgery was performed, and both legs were put in casts. He has not been able to play any sports since except golf.

> For the second Sunday in a row I was not able to go to church because Jeanette was not doing well. (March 21)
> Jeanette had fallen twice lately and had been eating less than she should for over a month, so Dr. Bibb wanted her to voluntarily go to Red River Hospital again to get her medications regulated. She agreed and went back the next day. (March 22)
> After not being on my trike for a month because of bad weather and staying close to Jeanette, I got back on it this afternoon and had a good 43-minute ride. The weather was perfect. Perry [Yancey] took me up to see Jeanette this evening. (March 30)
> Keith Lande took me to see Jeanette this evening. His little Allyson was with him. For Jeanette I had a carton of Dr Pepper and eight bananas. She was delighted when she saw the treats. She ate all of the bananas during the visit. I couldn't get much out of her in conversation. About 7 p.m. I kissed her goodbye. (Friday, April 2)
> David took me to see Jeanette this afternoon. I brought along a book Ron had given me two years ago. The title is Baseball's Fifty Greatest Games and I thought David might enjoy reading it while waiting for me. Jeanette ate the large Snicker bar and drank the Dr Pepper that I had brought, and I drank some Gatorade. I told her about my recent visit with Ralph Piper at Braum's. (April 3)
> After breakfast I began working on another marimba program which I hope to have Friday

night. I only played four songs when my foot hurt so much I had to sit down. Later I talked to Jeanette on the phone and she was in good spirits and talked more. She could hear better too. I practiced some more after supper and got the rest of the songs done. (April 7)

This is my 68th birthday and the first one without Jeanette in our five-year marriage. This evening when I entered her room, much to my surprise Jeanette was sitting in the chair instead of the bed. I was pleased to find her pleasant as she smiled when I came in. She gave me some good news. Dr. Bibbs said she might go home next week. I sure hope it is the first of the week. We had a good, long visit and the visiting hours were ending. We kissed and said goodbye. (April 8)

Shelby had experienced five years of his long-awaited female companionship in his sixty-eight years of life.

At this time, Ron was employed as minister of administration at Jersey Village Baptist Church with assets exceeding $15 million. Rod was CEO and part owner of M&M Manufacturing, which was steadily growing in plant square footage, number of employees, and revenue.

* * * * *

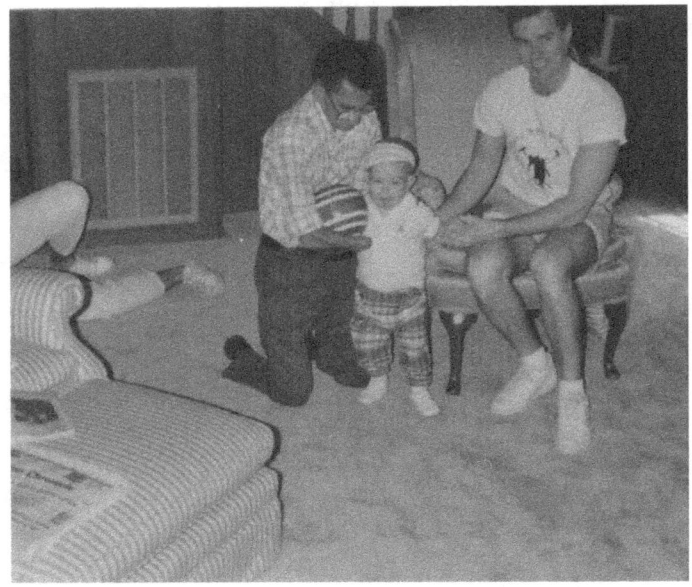

Shelby playing ball with Brandon a few days after his first birthday in March, 1991.

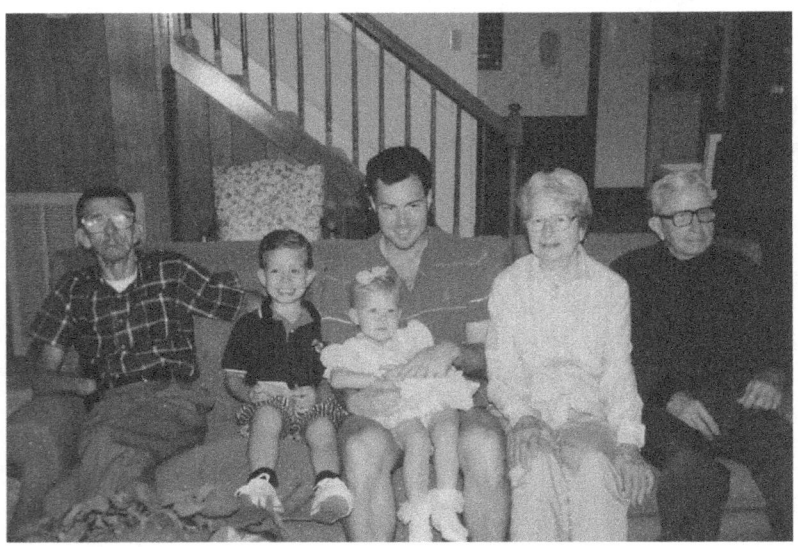

Shelby, Mother, and Dad visiting in Ron and Jeane's home in Jersey Village, TX in May of 1994. Ron Alan, Brandon, and Brittany lived next door.

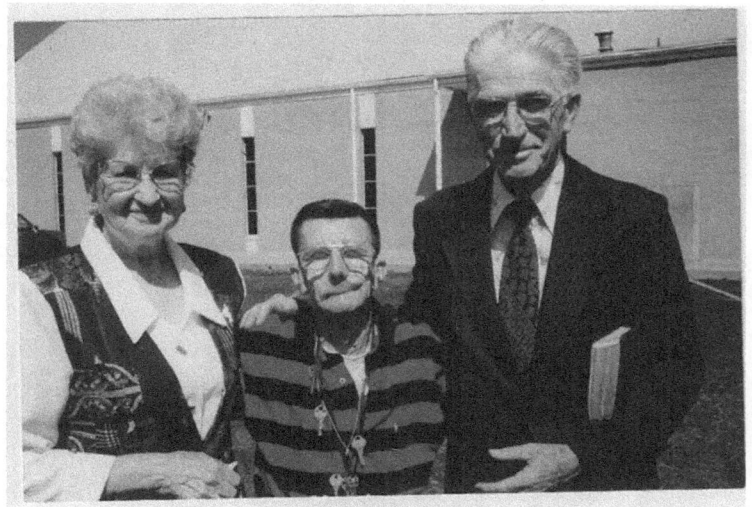

Aunt Almeda "Sis" and Uncle Isaac "Ike" join Shelby after worship at Trinity Baptist Church in Wichita Falls in 1997.

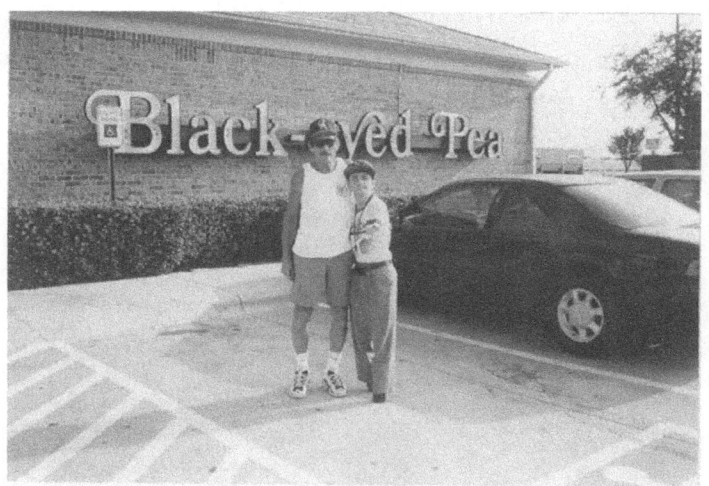

Jerry Allen and Shelby going to lunch before a Texas Ranger game on July 2, 1998. Rita took the photo.

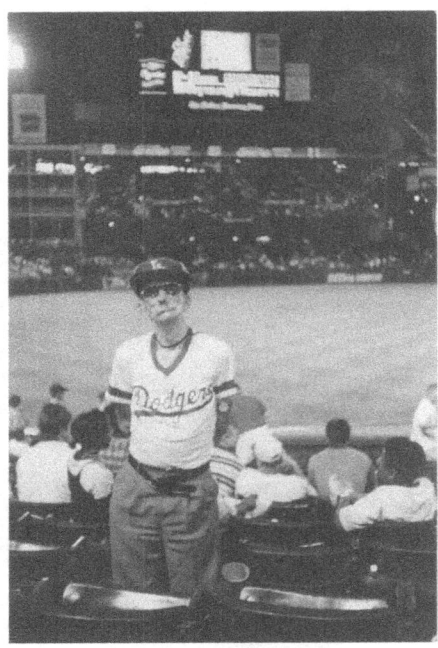

Shelby enjoying the Texas Ranger game in Arlington, Texas, dressed in his "obnoxious" Dodger uniform.

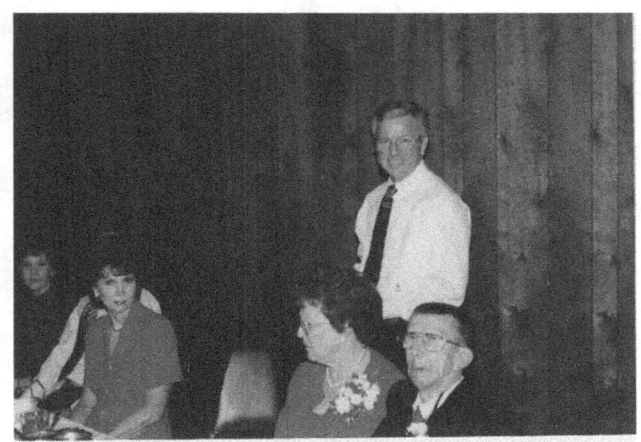

Wedding Reception on February 14, 1999.
(L-R: Jeane, Jeanette, Ron, Shelby)

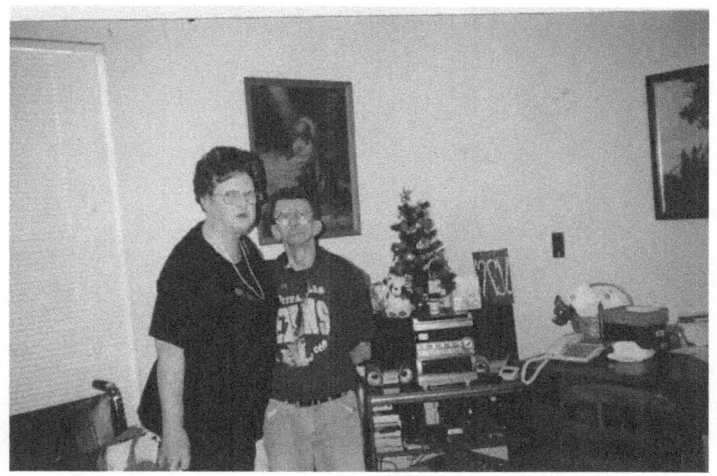

First Christmas after marriage.

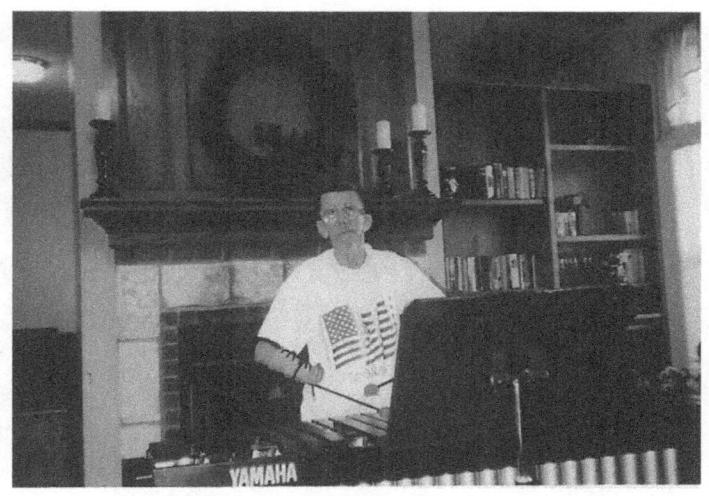

Shelby is practicing for another "An Evening in Marimba Land" on July 4, 2000.

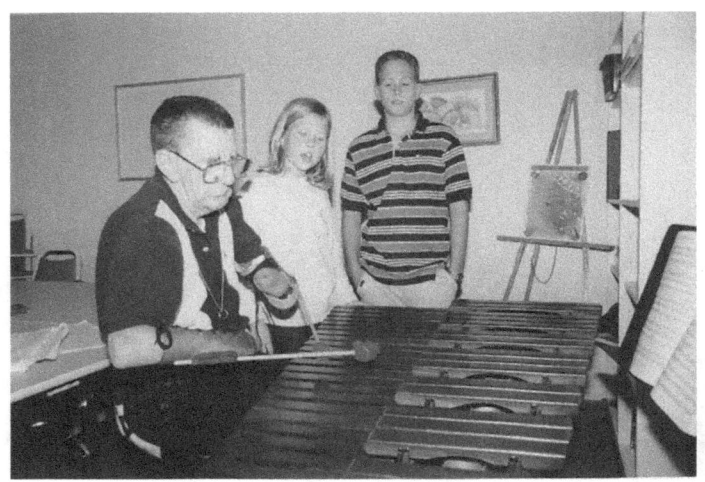

Brittany and Brandon watching Shelby practice on November 7, 2002.

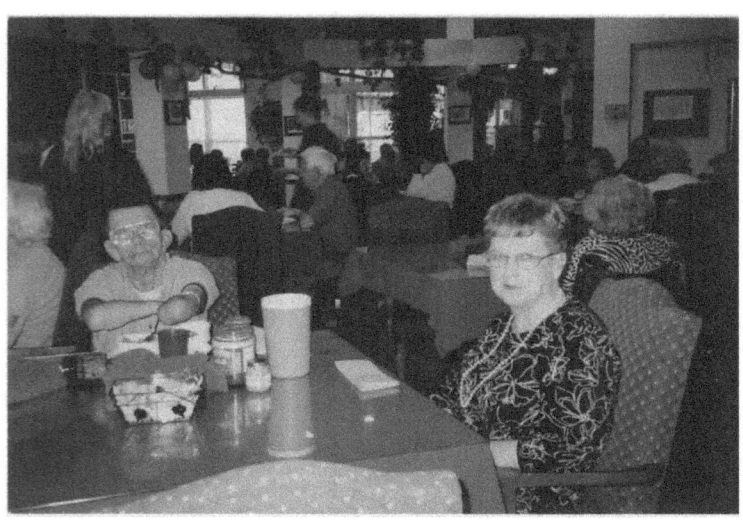

Shelby and Jeanette at lunch in Sterling House in 2003.

AN INCREDIBLE BOY AND A REMARKABLE MAN

United States after publication in 1930 by Platt & Munk. The story is used to teach children the value of optimism and hard work.

1. Go to Appendix C.
2. Go to Appendix C.
3. See Veron Seay in Appendix D.
4. A ski slope with a black diamond rating is said to be one of the more difficult slopes relative to others around it. When considering ski run categories, this 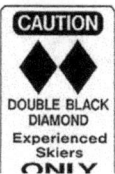 symbol has traditionally been used for the most difficult, though in recent years a double black diamond designation has been implemented. No matter if it is a single or double, however, it will still be one of the more difficult trails at a particular resort. A ski slope rated as a black diamond will often be one of the steepest on the hill. It may also be narrower than most of the other trails, requiring more frequent hairpin turns to control speed and positioning. Hazards may include cliffs, moguls (small bumps), trees, and rocks. A double black diamond course is sometimes even substantially more difficult than a single, and these courses may have extremely steep slopes and often are not groomed. It is up to the skier to traverse the mountain in a responsible way,

CHAPTER 8

Final Year: Sixty-Eight (2004–5)

Travis took me to see Jeanette who was sitting in a chair [Shelby had been encouraging her to sit up instead of lying down most of the time at Red River Hospital] when I got to her room. A smile once again was on her face as she happily greeted me, "Hello Shelby." Seeing she didn't have a Dr Pepper or cup of ice, I went to the nurses' station and asked for them. While Jeanette drank her Dr Pepper and I drank some coffee that I had brought, I told her the church choir would be doing an Easter Cantata tomorrow morning and that I would be playing "The Old Rugged Cross Made the Difference" for the offertory. After our visit of one hour and fifteen minutes, I told her goodbye with a kiss and departed. (Saturday, April 10, 2004)

On Easter morning at the worship service, I played during the offertory and then the choir presented a cantata titled "Worthy of the Lamb." In the four years that I have been a member of Trinity Baptist Church, this was the best I have heard the choir sing for an Easter or Christmas Cantata. It was splendid! [Shelby went on for two pages describing the scenes and drama that were presented during the cantata.] After the service I asked Perry [Yancey] to take me to Long John Silvers to get some shrimp for Jeanette. He took me to get six shrimp and then to RRH. Just like a woman, never satisfied, Jeanette said she wished I had brought some chips too. After my visiting time was up, I kissed her and said goodbye. (April 11)

To my surprise, Uncle Ike never came to move in here at Sterling House. I wonder if he has changed his mind. (April 12)

Uncle Isaac "Ike" Ewing died on May 7, 2004, at the age of eighty-three. Ron and Jeane attended the funeral at Lunn Funeral Home, and Shelby was a pallbearer. Shelby lost one of his favorite uncles, and now all his uncles were gone.

This afternoon I went with Jeanette for her appointment with Dr. Lucy Tan. She told Dr. Tan that she was having headaches and no appetite. Dr. Tan told her the headaches were caused by too much medication. She said that she could not stop the medications, but she could prescribe medicine to improve her appetite. (Monday, August 9)

Today Jeanette should find out when her cataract surgery will be scheduled. We went to Dr. Jeffery Harrington's office where she underwent many eye exams, and she answered many questions. The surgery was scheduled for August 31. (August 10)

This morning Perry took me to Callfield Boot & Shoe Repair to get my old pair of shoes repaired. The left shoe was twisted, the right shoe needed some sewing along the [metal] stave, and both shoes needed new soles. Also, I thought both shoes needed some cork [padding for the bottom of his stubs] put in them. I told Gaylon that I would pay for the repairs because I was tired of fooling around with the government and Health Pro [for approval]. Gaylon reminded me that we determined that the blue gel pads were better than cork. He said that the shoes would be ready in several days.

On the way home I asked Perry to stop at Braun's to drink some coffee. He went to Braun's and we each drank a cup and a half. I insisted on paying and did. (Tuesday, August 17)

About 1:30 p.m. Jeanette and I were lying down having our daily afternoon rest when the phone rang. I got up and answered it. On the line was Janet at Callfield Boot & Shoe Repair. She said that my shoes were ready. (Friday, August 20)

A Brotherhood breakfast was held in the Fellowship Hall this morning. Some of the men cooked eggs, sausage, gravy, biscuits, and tortillas. Travis grinded up some of all but tortillas for me. It turned out delicious to me. (Sunday, August 22)

This was the last entry from the diaries of Shelby that Ron was able to find. On August 31, Ron resigned from his job at Jersey Village Baptist Church and started his retirement. He and Jeane soon drove to Wichita Falls and visited family and friends. Shelby was not happy, and he complained about not being able to sleep well because Jeanette stayed up messing with rearranging clothes in the closet and other unnecessary late-at-night activities. He said nothing about any health issues except his right shoulder. Ron told him he needed to get a colonoscopy, but Shelby would not promise to do it.

Jeanette had a successful removal of her cataracts, but she continued to have health issues and periods of depression. Shelby and Jeanette began to have marital issues because of their ailments and their different sleep patterns. Shelby's right shoulder function was useless for playing his marimba, which was a big negative for him. He played his marimba less and less. Neither could look to the other for comfort and loving companionship. In November of 2004, Shelby began to experience discomfort in his lower abdomen. Dr. Tan tried to get him to have a colonoscopy, but he refused.

In mid-January of 2005, David called Ron and told him that Shelby was not in good shape, had lost a lot of weight, looked real pale, and refused to go to Dr. Tan. Ron and Jeane drove to Wichita Falls, and when they saw Shelby, they were very disturbed. Ron got some information from the staff at Sterling House, and then they took Shelby to ER at the Bethania Hospital.

While waiting with Shelby in the emergency room, a man in his forties asked Ron who was the man sitting next to him, and Ron said, "He's my brother, Shelby Stepp." The man acknowledged that he now remembered Shelby's name and that he first saw him at a dance hall where he had gone with an uncle when he was eight years old. He then said when he was eighteen that he saw Shelby there again dancing with women. Shelby heard the conversation, but he did not say anything. In Shelby's presence a few days later, Ron told David and Steve with levity what the man had said. Shelby interrupted by saying, "It was the Ponderosa!" Ron asked him jokingly if Mother knew he had gone there, and he quickly and loudly replied, "No." Then he paused and said, "And Daddy didn't either."

After some examinations and tests, Shelby was diagnosed with cancer of the liver. The doctor said that the cancer started in Shelby's colon. Shelby was admitted to the hospital. Several days later, Ron was told that the prognosis for Shelby was that his liver cancer was terminal, and the best thing for him was hospice care and medication for pain during his last weeks. Ron made the arrangements for Shelby to be moved to Hospice Center of Wichita Falls to receive the necessary care prescribed by the doctors. He was soon moved to University Park Manor (UPM), which provided him with a private room.

Ron's recent retirement was timely as it enabled Ron and Jeane to spend most of their time with Shelby in his last six weeks. They also were able to visit Ruth Franklin often because she was also in UPM. Ron and Jeane always enjoyed their visits with Ruth, and Ruth enjoyed them too. Ruth was the mother of Howard who was one of Ron's teammates on the Greyhounds and Broncos kid baseball teams, and Shelby was their batboy for two seasons.

Shelby was given good care at UPM and never experienced much pain.

While in the hospital and in hospice from January 21 to February 23, Shelby averaged eleven visitors each day with a high of nineteen visitors. He enjoyed the visitors until the last two days. On February 23, Shelby asked Ron if he could have some chili. Ron drove to Casa Manana downtown, which was Shelby's favorite Mexican food restaurant and ordered one bowl of chili. When Shelby got it, he was not able to eat much of it. Late that evening, Shelby asked, "Ron, will I see a bright light at the moment I die?" Ron answered that he would because he would see Jesus who said that he is the "Light of the world." The purpose of this response was to remind Shelby that he would see Jesus the instant the darkness of physical death came over him. *A comforting thought for a Christian facing death.*

Early the following morning, Ron received a call from the University Park Manor office informing him that Shelby showed signs that death would come soon. Ron called David and Steve, but

Steve did not answer. Ron, Jeane, and David arrived at UPM around 6:00 a.m. Ron and David began talking to Shelby, but they did not get much response. After a short period, Shelby looked up into Ron's eyes showing recognition and tried to speak. Ron took hold of Shelby's right stub, and David took hold of his left stub. If Steve had been there, he would have been stroking Shelby's brow, but Jeane still had not been able to contact Steve. Then Shelby's breathing became shallower, then the death rattle, and soon his breathing ceased. David immediately cried uncontrollably. Shelby stopped breathing at 7:50 a.m. and was officially pronounced dead at 8:20 a.m. In the moment Shelby took his last breath, *God gave him a perfect, whole, complete, heavenly body and said, "Shelby, you have fought the good fight, you have finished the race, you have kept the faith. Well done, my good and faithful servant, come and make music!"*

Ron and David began calling family and friends with the news of Shelby's death. Then they began arrangements for the funeral service to be held two days later. Shelby's obituary and funeral notice were given to the *Wichita Falls Times Record News*. The visitation and funeral service were scheduled with Owens & Brumley Funeral Home, and interment would be at one of Daddy's gravesites at Crestview Memorial Park. Ron was asked to be interviewed about Shelby's life at the KFDX-TV Channel 3 station on the Seymour Highway. Ron went for the interview that afternoon. The theme of what Ron shared about Shelby was that he lived for Jesus, inspired thousands to do their best at all times, under all circumstances, and to give God the glory for all their service to others. The recording session went well, but it was aired Friday evening while Shelby's visitation was underway. Most of the family and friends most interested in Shelby missed the interview.

The visitation was well attended as was the funeral service. At the former, many family and friends shared what an inspiration Shelby was to them. For some, it had been a lifetime of inspiration. At the latter event, Ron had placed one of Shelby's marimbas at the front with his newest pair of shoes sitting on his Bible on top of the marimba. Beside the Bible were Shelby's newest cuffs with mallets. Ron also placed at the front a photo album Mother had put together of Shelby's photos from babyhood to middle adulthood. Also, several documents including his short biography written by Ron,[1] his salvation experience that he wrote in 1992, Mother's article about Shelby, a letter from Shelby to Rod, and a letter from Shelby to Ron. Pallbearers were the six Stepp boys.

During the funeral service, Rod delivered a humorous and touching eulogy.[2] Then Ron delivered a tribute to Shelby and a challenge to Christians in attendance. He spoke extemporaneously, but late that evening, he wrote from memory what he had said.[3]

After the funeral, many shared with the Stepp boys what Shelby had meant to them and how he had inspired them.

Shelby Ray "Poofus" Stepp was laid to rest at 12:30 p.m. on Saturday, February 26, 2005, in Grave 3, Block 6, in the Garden of Devotion Section of Crestview Memorial Park of Wichita Falls, Texas. His monument is shown below.

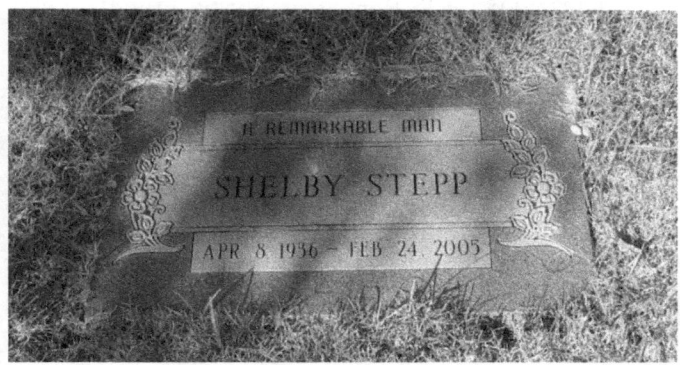

This long-awaited story of Shelby Ray "Poofus" Stepp comes to an end. But only the written text of his story ends here. *His story* is now *history* and will be handed down generation to generation by the Stepp family and many other families because it is a Christian story of living for Jesus with hope, courage, commitment, determination, perseverance, humility, a healthy sense of humor, and love. Jesus said we show our love for him by loving and serving others. Shelby did that more consistently than anyone I know other than Mother.

The end.

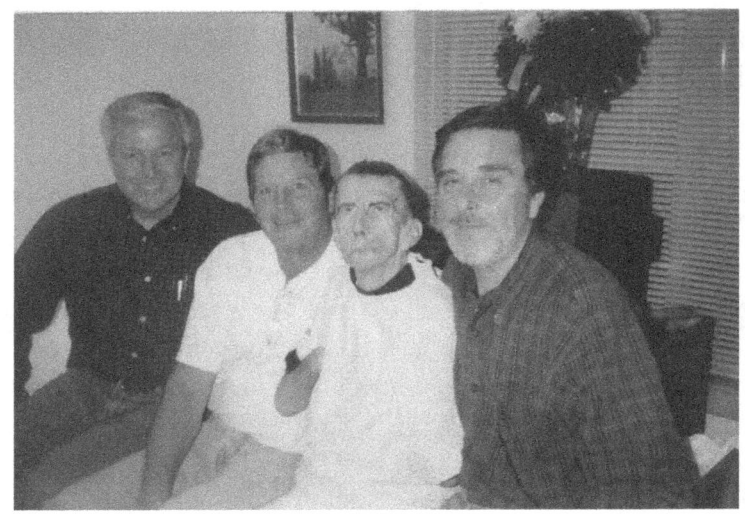

Photo of Shelby taken on Mother's birthday Feb. 11, 2005. (L-R: Ron, Steve, Shelby, David)

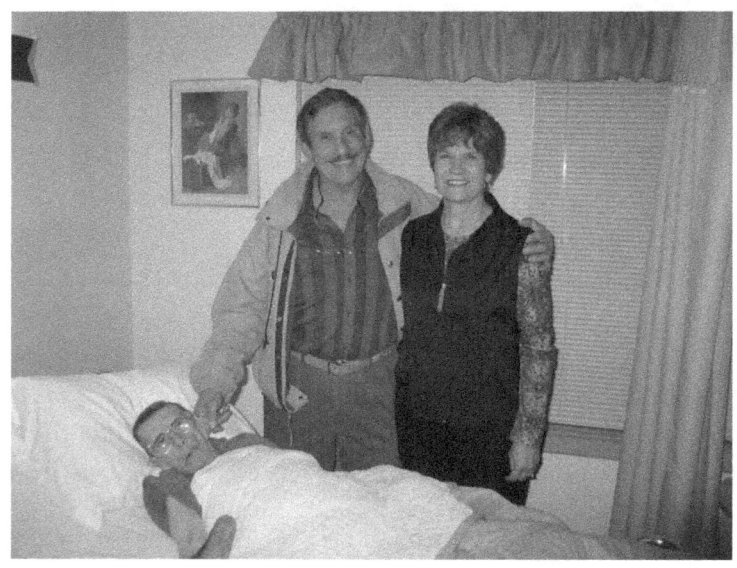

Last photo taken of Shelby on February 18, 2005, with good friends, Jerry and Rita Allen.

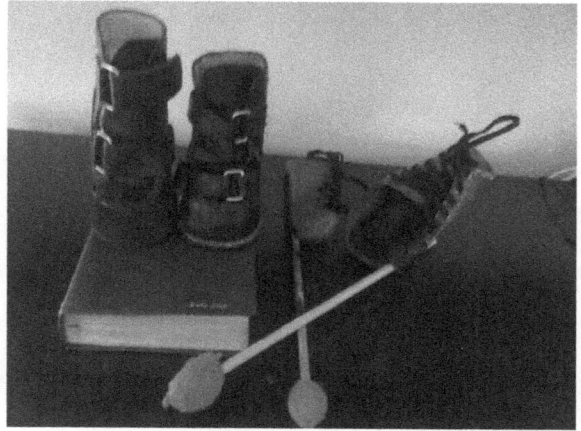

Shelby's Bible, shoes, cuffs and mallets as displayed at his funeral service.

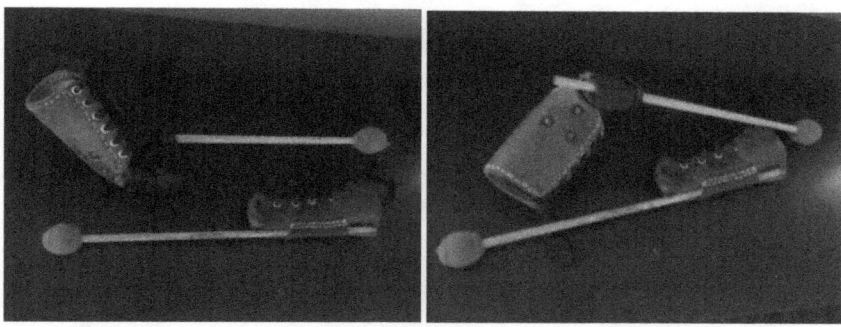

Shelby's cuffs with mallets front view   Cuffs with mallets backside view

---

and those attempting a difficult slope who are not ready for it are subjecting themselves to risk of serious injury.
1. Go to Appendix B.
2. Go to Appendix B.
3. Go to Appendix B.

APPENDIX

APPENDIX A

Testimonials

From Stella Jo Ewing Stepp, March 12, 1991:

The oldest of four boys, Shelby was always accepted as one of the boys when he was growing up. He was not like a handicap, but always went along with the group.

Not beginning school until he was ten years old, Shelby was reading books himself within eight weeks. Two years later he had already reached the fifth grade.

Shelby had the honor of walking across the stage graduating with his class of 1956 seniors from Wichita Falls Senior High. He continued to attend school at Draughon's Business College in Wichita Falls, made good grades and received diplomas in accounting and bookkeeping.

Shelby is talented in music and he began playing the marimba at age fifteen. He currently plays at Highland Heights Baptist Church where he is a member, and he plays for nursing homes and clubs.

From Ronald Lee Stepp, June 17, 2021:

Shelby's primary objective in life from age twelve to his final days was to be the boy and man that God purposed him to be. It included putting the other person first. It meant pulling for the underdog and helping the underprivileged. It also meant relying on

God for the strength and ability to do what needed to be done in the name of Jesus Christ. Finally, Shelby desired that all glory due for what he did for others be given to God.

Ron's last reflections on his relationship with Shelby and how he misses him today (Feb. 10, 2021):

- Shelby was dependent on Mother and others all his life.
- He did the best he could every day and was positive about receiving help with what he could not do.
- God wants us to be dependent on Him for what we cannot do that should be done.
- He also wants us to do the best we can and be positive about receiving His help for the rest of what needs to be done.
- David, Rod, Butch, Jim, and Steve miss helping Shelby and cutting up with him and talking to him about life. Our family reunions are infrequent now because of Shelby's absence.
- I was probably more inspired by Shelby than anyone because of our close relationship during our first eighteen years together. Except for Mother and Thelma Williams Lucas Thompson, I influenced Shelby more than anyone. Those were our most formative years.
- Writing Shelby's story has given me a deeper understanding of Shelby, a broader appreciation of his accomplishments, and a more thankful heart for God mercifully calling Shelby home when He did. Shelby would have been greatly challenged to live abundantly without serving God by playing his marimba. God promises to never give us more of a burden than we can bear.
- Shelby will always be active in my life. He is very real to me today."

From Mary Weatherford Mock, February 28, 2005:

I remember Shelby from my childhood. My family shopped at the store on Grant Street daily. I was in town today visiting my parents, who are at Texhoma Christian Care Center, when my sister told me about Shelby's passing. I'm so sad even though I haven't seen him in years. He was truly remarkable.

He was 12 years older than my sister and me, but he was our friend. We loved the music he played at our church Highland Heights (Baptist). He had a beautiful handwriting and a great sense of humor. We didn't see Shelby as different—he was special. I was proud to know him and glad to read in the paper he had a wonderful life. He will be missed by so many.

Shelby is with God now, but he'll be in our hearts forever.
Mary Weatherford Mock
Daughter of Melvin & Oleta Weatherford who lived at 2507 Buchanan.

From Joe Hallford, April 23, 2020:

Please be gracious in accepting my feeble attempt to remember such a man as Shelby and the Stepp family. Be mindful of what a very minuscule & infinitesimal role I played in the life in question. If measured in time our relationship would score very low over the years, but if measured by the quality of Shelby's influence on my life it is great.

Shelby Stepp was a most interesting person in that he stood tall in his little shoes and faced life as the Captain of his ship. He knew what he believed and no matter what life threw at him, he never wavered in that faith and unwavering devotion to his family and his God. Shelby truly cared about life from his as well as our perspectives. He was filled with love.

Shelby was a remarkable friend and person in how he took what he was given and made the most of it. He talked when they said he wouldn't, he walked when they said he wouldn't, he went to school when they said he couldn't, he played the marimba when they said he couldn't, he kept box/line scores of baseball games as accurately as anyone, he composed music and played the piano with no hands or fingers, he walked all over Wichita Falls taking care of business without assistance because he knew he could. Remarkable? Yes, and I could go on and on.

Admirable? I don't know anyone who really knew Shelby who didn't admire him, his values, his dedication and devotion to his family, his church and mankind in general. It might have raised an eyebrow or two and even made the paper…but how can you not admire someone for throwing a rock at a woman who was mistreating a dog!? Admirable? You're darn tootin!

I can honestly say (and I know I am prejudiced) but I can think of nothing regarding Shelby Stepp that was less than honorable. Perhaps there are those that might have *heard* something about Shelby like visiting a dance hall or the like…but I venture to guess, if anyone perceives that as less than admirable, they were *not there to see him* or they would not think less of him…maybe even more. Where did Jesus walk?

Shelby got a late start and played catch up the rest of his life. Unfortunately, because of our prejudices and lack of confidence he never fully caught up. But Shelby ran the race and never quit trying no matter how many times he was knocked down. He continued to get up, brush himself off and get back in the race. Many people probably thought Shelby's life was hell. Those of us who knew him know that he lived in heaven on earth. He didn't do it by preaching, although he could do that, but by living as an example of how to face adversity. Kites rise against, not with, the wind.

If you look perseverance up in the dictionary you should see a picture of Shelby Ray Stepp holding a baseball bat teaching kids to play ball. Oh yes, he did! No doubt! To quote *People Magazine*, "Stubby wants no help,"

The handicap that angered or troubled me the most throughout my life with Shelby was people's inability or unwillingness to communicate with him. Shelby had a good mind and was a problem solver but was never given a chance to prove it. I would hope if Shelby entered the world today, he would be allowed to contribute more because of our attitudes toward differences in people. There was no reason Shelby could not have held a full-time job of significance using his abilities and intelligence. He could have made a greater contribution to society and some small business were it not for prejudices. Although he and I never discussed this and I tried to conceal my anger over it…if he had any, I never picked up on it because that would have gone against his Christian principles. When I picture him on his hands and knees hoeing weeds in August at Highland Heights (Baptist Church), it saddens me that he wasn't allowed to do more. Yet I am thankful that Highland Heights gave him a job. He was thankful, that was Shelby. That's why he was bigger than me.

I can't remember life without Shelby. He was there in my earliest memories. There was probably not a family closer to my family than Shelby's family. Some of us were at the other's house daily… many times before sunup in our underwear. David was my best friend and the only brother I ever had. As kids do, we sometimes had our differences. One day I had David down on the ground and suddenly a hailstorm erupted from above. It was Shelby giving me what I deserved with both nubs. I jumped up and ran as fast as I could across two streets and five houses to get home. Our porch had five steps up to the front porch. Only because Shelby had to get down and crawl up those steps did I get away. I ran in, locked the screen door, and went to hide. Shelby knocked on the door and told Faye (that was my mother) I had to come out and we had to sit and talk about it all. But you know what? Shelby forgave me and never held it against me. That's the mark of a very tall man with big shoes to fill.

Adjectives to describe Shelby: strong, persevering, courageous, committed, kind, thoughtful, peaceful, warm, and humble.

Lessons younger people might learn from Shelby are to try and not say "I can't do that" He could hit a baseball with the best of 'em. He could play the piano; He could catch a ball and throw a ball or a rock with accuracy. He could eat, talk, and sing…you try any or all of that without hands, feet, or a tongue. But he didn't say "can't"…he tried and succeeded because of his attitude and efforts.

Shelby was surrounded by good people who were not only his role models but those of so many of us lucky enough to grow up in the Sam Houston School vicinity during the 1940s and 50s. These were strong people of character who led their lives with compassion and love for one another. Shelby's parents were truly people we looked up too, loved, and respected.

I heard it said that when Shelby was born the doctors wanted to put him over there in the corner. That's what they did in those days. Stella said "No! He has as much right to live as anyone else! Do whatever you can for him." That is strength and courage in the face of adversity. You know kites rise against, not with the wind? Oh! I said that already, but it is true and so appropriate when you think of what challenges Stella was willing to face for the love of a son. For the Love of a Son… I read about that in the Bible.

Shelby's code of life or conduct was to care deeply for man and life. It was religious based, from his being brought up and committed to Christianity. Shelby was baptized on Easter Sunday when he was twelve. I dare say Shelby's loving heart was already in place when he made that commitment. Shelby was a child of God in all that he did because kindness was the center of his soul. Shelby cared. Six years later I followed in Shelby's footsteps on Easter Sunday at Highland Heights. I was eight. He led the way.

Shelby was my hero. There were a couple if items (in the questionnaire Ron sent to family and friends) I did not respond to simply because I am not worthy to stand in judgement of Shelby. I don't know how tall Shelby was, but he towered over me. I stood in his shadow and not he in mine. With God's grace we all learned something powerful and humble from our dear friend.

Each of us and the world is a better place because Shelby was here and touched our lives. During a brief theological discussion Shelby said to me he would be sad in a way when he got to Heaven because it was his understanding that we would have different forms and he would not recognize his mother. I pray Shelby recognized Stella and is "dancing," yes, I said dancing with the angels as we try to shine a light on his life.

Thank you, Shelby…for everything you gave.

From Jim Booher, April 27, 2020:

Shelby, lovingly called Poofus, was interesting to all of us kids because he was different. He was just a part of the neighborhood gang. He did have limitations, but we all knew that and made concessions as needed. I think all of us were careful to make sure other people who did not know him were informed about who he was and his limitations in no uncertain terms, if need be!

Since he was two months older than me, and we attended the same church, we grew up together. My family moved to Avenue Q when I was four, so he was always a part of my life until I left for college in 1954.

As we grew up in childhood, I was impressed with his abilities of running, writing, playing catch with a ball, batting a ball, and communicating in his writings. His speech was the biggest handicap in his life with others. He became an inspiration to me and untold thousands of other people.

I have never known of anyone who has overcome as many handicaps as Shelby did. I have counted it an honor to tell a lot of people throughout my life about Shelby and what he overcame. Determined, persistent, tenacious, loving, and remarkable best describe his character. His determination to succeed despite all the odds handed him at birth made him remarkable.

The only thing about Shelby close to being negative was that he sure could hurt you with a jab with one of his stubs!

He had a sharp mind, good music talent, and a willingness to share himself with others. All his talents were given by God.

I am so disappointed now that I did not have a relationship with Shelby in our adult years. If I would have only taken a little time when I was visiting my parents in Iowa Park,[1] to have stopped by to visit him. That is my loss!

From Bill McFall on May 20, 2020:

In 1943 when I was six years old, Dad bought me a used bicycle, hard to find because of the war effort, from Bobby Hall. One early morning as I was venturing from my Tilden Street refuge exploring my newfound freedoms, I decided to ride by Bobby Hall's residence.[2]

---

[1] Iowa Park is thirteen miles west of Wichita Falls.
[2] Bobby Hall's backyard on Cumberland Avenue was adjacent to Shelby's backyard on Grant Street.

As I turned off Grant Street onto Cumberland Avenue, I passed a gas station[3] where a number of people were gathered. As I gazed at the crowd, my eyes fell upon a shocking sight, a boy with no hands, no feet, and a barely discernable mouth, sitting on the soft drink box. The sight hit me like I had been knocked from my bicycle. I was so saddened by the sight of that poor boy that I rode home crying.

Five years later in the sixth grade, Crockett School played Sam Houston School in touch football and softball. At those games, I met Ron and Rod Stepp, and others who would become my friends. To my surprise, there was that poor, physically disabled boy acting as a batboy, cheering on his team, and acting like a preteen. I met Ron's brother Shelby. I learned that Shelby was an intelligent, personable, and active youth who participated in the same activities as the other kids he was around. I was amazed to see him run on the stubs where there should have been feet to catch a ball in a glove on a stub where there was no hand, discard the glove and throw the ball with both stubs. When batting he would grasp the bat between his forearms, take a full swing with that incomplete body, and after hitting the ball which he often did, pumping those little stub feet like pistons as he scurried around the bases. He cheered and danced in jubilation whenever he or a teammate scored a run or made a good play.

In time I made the transition from pity and sadness to amazement and admiration over how Shelby with so many limitations, enjoyed life, inspired others with his accomplishments, and gave others a reason to be thankful for their blessings.

I did not have contact with Shelby during the next few years until I was in high school and began dating Janice Hallford. She and Ron Stepp were close friends for years and Shelby was a regular visitor in the Hallford residence. I learned more about his intelligence, his endearing personality, and the respect he had earned from all who knew him. He even earned the love and respect of the woman Rod said was "the meanest woman in the world," Faye Hallford, Janice's mother! I guess Shelby came to like and respect me because of the

---

[3] The gas station was owned and operated by Chester Hallford at that time. Chester would later become Bill's father-in-law. Was Shelby a matchmaker?

relationship I had developed with Faye, Janice, and Ron, because as our relationship grew, he would wrap those stubby arms around me in greeting and departing.

Shelby Stepp was one of the positive great influences of my life in helping me learn that God has a purpose for everyone, and Shelby inspired people to be all they could be no matter what the obstacles and limitations might be.

May God continue to bless his soul!

From Mickey Aboussie, January 6, 2021:

Ron, the most common thing that reminds me of Shelby was his sense of humor and ability to laugh at himself. He would chuckle at almost any kind of story you told him and could REMEMBER the story long after you told it. He really appreciated the fact that his friends loved him, and he shared everything in his possession to convince them to laugh with him, not at him. He was a neighborhood treasure. Once his name came up, all other discussion items faded, and we all joined in to recall Shelby stories. His vision was poor but he could see right through you, if you dared to be obtuse about an important subject. He loathed politics and would not talk about the President or Congress easily. He would say Washington was a "joke." Despite his physical limitations, he loved to play catch with either a football or baseball. And he would come to any game played by his friends, at any time and place. He was tireless in walking with you and just chatting about really nothing. He just wanted to be loved and appreciated and he indeed was…in spades. I can never remember a moment when he was critically unfair about anybody or anything. His ability to talk freely about people, events or ideas was limitless. His was a simple world, with simple speech and ideas. But to this day, I remember him so fondly, it hurts my heart that he is no longer with us.

APPENDIX B

Documents

Letter from Joe Hallford to Ron, David, and Steve, February 24, 2005

Dear Ron, David, and Steve

Today[4] Heaven is a little brighter. We mourn at our loss of Shelby, but think what a blessed picnic he had today.

I recently volunteered to deliver the devotionals for a group at our church. One of them seems appropriate for today. The author is unknown.

A stranger came by the other day with an offer that set me to thinking. He wanted to buy my old barn that sits out by the road. In a friendly way, I told him upfront that he was crazy. He was a city type. You could tell by his clothes, his car, his hands, and the way he talked. He said he was driving by and saw that beautiful barn sitting out there in the tall grass and wanted to know if it was for sale. I told him he had a funny idea of beauty. Sure, it was a handsome building in its day, but there's been a lot of winters pass with their snow and ice and howling wind. The summer sun's beat down

---

[4] Shelby died on February 24, 2005.

on that old barn until all the paint's gone, and the wood has turned silver and gray. Now the old building leans a good deal, looking kind of tired. Yet, that fellow called it beautiful.

That set me to thinking. I walked out to the field and just stood there, gazing at that old barn. The stranger said he planned to use the lumber to line the walls of his den in a new country home he's building down the road. He said you couldn't get paint that beautiful. Only years of standing out in the weather, bearing the storms and scorching sun, only that can produce beautiful barn wood.

It came to me then. We're a lot like that, you and I. Only it is on the inside that the beauty grows with us. Sure, we turn silver and gray too, and lean a bit more than we did when we were young and full of sap. But the Good Lord knows what He is doing. And as the years pass, He's busy using the hard wealth of our lives, the dry spells and the stormy seasons, to do a job beautifying our souls that nothing else can produce. And to think how often folks holler because they want life to be easy!

They took the old barn down today and hauled it away to beautify a rich man's house. And I reckon someday you and I will be hauled off to Heaven to take on whatever chores the Good Lord has for us on the Great Sky Ranch. And I suspect we will be more beautiful for the seasons we have been through here, and just maybe add a bit of beauty to our Father's house.

> Think with me of the many storms Shelby weathered for 68 years. No barn wood can compare. He will truly brighten Heaven's Gate and all that dwells within.
>
> May today there be peace within you. May you trust God that you are exactly where you are meant to be. I believe that friends are quiet Angels who lift us to our feet when our wings have trouble remembering how to fly. Shelby has done that for each of us.

RONALD STEPP

    Thank God for Shelby Stepp and thank Shelby for being my friend.
    May God hold you in the palm of His hand.

Love,
Joe Hallford

Eulogy for Shelby Stepp by Rod Stepp, February 26, 2005

I am Rod Stepp and Shelby's double cousin. Shelby and I had a lot in common:

- We had the same last name.
- Our mothers were sisters and best friends.
- Our dads were brothers and best friends and business partners—Stepp Brothers Grocery/Service Station/Café.
- We had the same four grandparents.
- We had the same cousins, aunts, and uncles.
- We celebrated the same birthday. I was born on his first birthday.
- We lived in the same house when we were born.
- We lived in the same duplex for the next seven years.
- Until I left for college, we lived within seven blocks except for 14 months we lived 12 blocks apart and in 1946 for six months Shelby lived in Hugo, Oklahoma, which was 210 miles away.
- During our early years of childhood, we played together every day along with his brother Ronnie.

Although we had a lot in common, there were several significant *Differences*. I had two hands, two feet, a mouth, and a normal tongue. He had no hands, no feet, no mouth, and a one-inch tongue.

These *Differences* were extreme during our first six years together, but not as extreme as they would be in later years. We played together, ate together, and went to church together.

But when Ronnie and I went to first grade, Shelby was left at home and the *Differences* grew larger. But Butch and Jim and David came along and eased the absence of Rod and Ronnie.

Then at age ten, Shelby got to enter public school grade one and he excelled in class. Again, the *Differences* seemed to be less than before. Shelby even rode to school with us.

But as we all grew up, and when Ronnie and I went off to college, the *Differences* became significant. Shelby realized that his life was going to be different from ours.

Let me stop and reflect for a moment:

- I do not think I ever heard Shelby complain about his plight.
- He must have paid attention to Brother Huff, the pastor at HHBC where we all attended as kids, in Vacation Bible School when he said at assembly every morning: *"I will do the best I can with what I have, and where I am."*

But Shelby never complained. He was energetic. He had a quick wit and liked a good joke and liked to get one up on you. He did the best he could with what he had—every day.

He had to be a pioneer—He had to blaze a new trail—and he did it very well, and with no complaints.

After I finished college, got married, was in the process of raising a family, and beginning a career, I selfishly forgot about the *Differences*.

Of course, I still saw Shelby at family events, but I was in my own world. I still forgot about the *Differences*, but Shelby reminded me of them in a letter that I would like to read to you in closing… This letter was written on Nov. 5, 1965. Shelby was 29 years old and I was 28.

Apparently, Mother had mentioned that Shelby had a new entertainment—he would visit a nightclub a few times each week. Either I was surprised and opposed to this, or my mom told Shelby that I was. I then received this letter from Shelby. The letter shows that Shelby remembered the *Differences*, and he was handling it in his own way. He had grown up.

November 5, 1965

Dear Rod,

    I am writing this letter to you for the sole purpose of answering the remarks you made about me going to a night club. I learned of this from your mother the other night while visiting, and I was a little disturbed about it.
    I have gone to this one particular night club called the Ponderosa about five times for one reason—and one reason only—and that was merely to sit and listen to live music from a rock and roll band. I do not indulge in any alcoholic beverages or sit at the same table with people who do. Therefore, I strongly feel that my hands are clean.
    I am going all out to make up for everything I missed in my younger years. You might say my wild oats are being sown late in life.
    I remember having to sit at home day in and day out while you and Ron went out and had a blast. It really did not bother me that much, but I wanted to mention it just to put you to thinking how lucky it is for a person to be physically normal and be able to do things you did.
    Let's go back to your college days at dear ole panty wanty A&M. Whenever parties were thrown, beer was always served. Of course, I know that you did not take the stuff, but you were there. Being at these parties, were you condoning sin? That's about what you are saying that I am doing.

Thus, there is no difference in me going to a night club and your going to those beer drinking parties.

May I kindly suggest that the next time you want to bark, make sure it is up the right tree.

Your cousin,
Shelby Stepp

Eulogy for Shelby Stepp by Ron Stepp,[5] February 26, 2005

If I was in Houston, I would introduce myself as Ron Stepp, but in Wichita Falls, I am Shelby Stepp's brother, Ronnie. Shelby has been full of surprises for me all his life. I didn't hear about his Ponderosa escapades that Rod just mentioned until the day six weeks ago when we admitted Shelby to the hospital where he was diagnosed with cancer. While waiting with Shelby in the emergency room, a man in his forties asked me who he was, and I said, "He's my brother, Shelby Stepp." The man acknowledged that he now remembered Shelby's name and that he first saw him at a dance hall where he had gone with an uncle when he was eight years old. He then said when he was eighteen that he saw Shelby there again dancing with women. In Shelby's presence a few days later, I told my brothers David and Steve with levity what the man had said. Shelby interrupted by saying, "It was the Ponderosa!" I asked him jokingly if Mother knew he had gone there, and he quickly and loudly replied, "No," paused and said, "and Daddy didn't either."

Another surprise that I learned about recently happened in 1960. Steve told me that when he was about five, he, David, and Shelby got in the '57 Chevy that Daddy had recently bought from me, and Shelby drove it off the church parking lot adjacent to their driveway and turned left onto York Street, turned left on Hayes Road, then left again at the alley, and back onto the parking lot. Steve said he was standing up in the seat while Shelby drove that route several

---

[5] Ron wrote this from memory that night while it was fresh on his mind. He thought it might be good to have some day.

times. David was in the middle of the front seat helping Shelby with the brakes. Shelby was twenty-four at that time, and I guess he just decided he was going to drive a car to show that he could.

When Shelby was eight, he got up on his stubs and walked for the first time, and he had the audacity to do it when I was not there. I had spent the night with Rod. It was probably the first time I had spent the night away from my family. When Rod and I walked to my house that Saturday morning, we were in for a very big surprise. Shelby could walk. Soon a local cobbler made him a pair of special shoes, and it wasn't long until Shelby was up and running.

I grew up with Shelby. My first remembrance of him is seeing him sitting inside our front screen door while Rod and I played outside. After he started walking, he played with us as cowboys and Indians, soldiers, and in sports. He learned to hit, throw, and catch a baseball; pass, catch, and kick a football; and shoot a regulation basketball through a regulation goal from inside the free throw line (making nine of ten was his best effort).

At age ten, Shelby started to public school with a special education teacher at Austin Elementary. He made two grades his first year and two grades his second year. That put him one grade behind me. I thought he was going to catch me and pass me! Shelby began to learn to play the marimba when he was fifteen. A few years later, my junior year in high school, he played his marimba and tap danced for the 1,800 students at WFSH. I was surprised because he and Mother had kept his program a secret from me. He finished twelve grades in ten years and graduated from Old High with the class of '56, just one behind me. He then went to Draughon's Business College and earned a diploma in accounting and bookkeeping.

Shelby began to apply for employment where he could use his sharp mind and business training. His handwriting was readable, and he operated a calculator by using the eraser-end of a lead pencil to punch the keys. After a while, it became obvious that the workplace was not ready to provide for an employee with his multiple handicaps. (It became obvious that his major handicap was his abnormal speech.) He sold papers for two years, worked at the Opportunity

Workshop checking out tools to the workers for five years, and then became assistant custodian at his church for most of his adult life. He was known for his hard work doing manual labor, even hoeing weeds on his knees instead of using his sharp mind.

Why did God choose to handicap Shelby so severely? I think it was because God knew what drive Shelby had and that he would be a "superman" bringing glory to him. By divine providence, Shelby was handicapped so that he could bring glory to God by inspiring others to be the best they could be. Shelby has been an inspiration to me all my sixty-seven years and still is.

I want us to focus now on the *legacy* that Shelby has left for us who are here today. This *legacy* is first to the six Stepp boys who remain. *Who's gonna fill those shoes?* (Pointing to Shelby's shoes prominently displayed on top of his Bible on his marimba). David and I donated Shelby's two marimbas to Old High this week. The band director at WFSH was very pleased, and he said several students would be very happy to get to use them.[6] One of those students may carry on Shelby's legacy in playing the marimba to inspire others. But *who's gonna fill those shoes?* Rod, will you? I don't think so. I know that I won't be able to fill Shelby's shoes. Maybe one of you here today can fill his shoes.

What qualifications are required to fill Shelby's shoes? There are two. The *first* is Philippians 4:13 NKJV, Shelby's favorite Bible verse*:* "I can do all things through Christ who strengthens me." I *can do… all* things…through *Christ*…who *strengthens* me. The *second* is found in Shelby's written Christian testimony:

One day after walking over to Aunt Ruby's house to visit, I paged through her Bible looking at the colored illustrations. Near the end of the Bible, I came to a picture of Jesus hanging on a cross. I studied the illustration for a while then hollered for Aunt Ruby to come

---

[6] In February 2021, Ron spoke with Justin Lewis, band director of Wichita Falls High School, about the use of Shelby's two marimbas. Justin said that they had been used annually by students in the band since 2005 and were much appreciated and especially helpful because of budget cuts to purchases of band instruments. He also said that the students have a practice of naming the school instruments and named the Ludwig marimba "Ginger."

explain something. I asked her what Jesus had done that was so bad that they did this terrible thing to Him? She told me that Jesus had done nothing wrong, but that He had to die for us so that each of us could have the opportunity to become a Christian. I asked her how I could become a Christian. She told me that if I believed that Jesus was the Son of God, that He gave His life in payment for my sins, that if I asked forgiveness for my sins, and asked Jesus to come into my heart and be my Savior and Lord; I would become a Christian. I believed and got on my knees and asked Jesus into my heart.

Soon after becoming a Christian, Shelby began to live for Jesus. In all things, *he did the best he could with what he had*. No obstacle was insurmountable. He truly believed that he could do all things because God would enable him. Down through these many years, Shelby has been an inspiration to many of all ages. He has served in his church and has entertained in many other churches, in nursing homes, and at Christian retreats. *Who's gonna fill those shoes?* Shelby would tell us that any of us can if we are a Christian who truly believes *"I can do all things through Christ who strengthens me." Who's gonna fill those shoes?* Rod, Butch, Jim, David, Steve (Shelby's three double cousins and other two brothers), the six of us could surely be used by God to fill Shelby's shoes. *We can…together.*

Shelby's life was a struggle from the first moment of birth, when he had to breathe without a mouth, to his last hour. But in contrast, his death was quick, quiet, painless, and peaceful. Early Thursday morning, he became unresponsive. I took hold of his right wrist stub, and David took hold of his left elbow stub. If Steve had been there, he would have been stroking Shelby's brow, but we had not been able to contact him. We told Shelby that we loved him. After a short period, he looked up into my eyes showing recognition and tried to speak. Then his breathing became shallower, and then, it ceased. He stopped breathing at 7:50 a.m. and was pronounced dead at 8:20 a.m. In the moment Shelby took his last breath, *God gave him a perfect, whole, complete, heavenly body, and God said, "Shelby, you have fought the good fight, you have finished the race, you have kept the faith. Well done, my good and faithful servant!"*

APPENDIX C

Anecdotes

- Ron and David do not remember ever seeing Shelby or Daddy cry. Ron does not remember crying himself until September 12, 1996, when Jeane told him that David had called and said that Mother had died.
- It was an honor to have known Shelby and been a small part of his life. Jerry and I loved and adored him. I can just see him laughing hard, stomping his feet, and slapping his legs! (Rita Allen)
- Cousin Terry Erwin remembers asking Shelby to attend a dinner party at his church and play his marimba. Shelby showed up in a white Elvis Presley outfit with a high collar and low V-neck exposing his chest. He played some Elvis songs, and the audience enjoyed his performance.
- No family member can remember when Shelby stopped sitting on the front row of a movie theater or when he stopped getting down on his knees when the scene became scary, but Ron thinks it was at about the age of eighteen for the former and sixteen for the latter.
- Also, no family member can remember when Shelby stopped doing his daily self-taught exercises, but Ron thinks it was in the late 1960s when his work at Opportunity Workshop and riding his trike replaced his exercise routine.

- Jeanette Averitt Stepp had no relationship with the Stepp family after Shelby's death. She did not attend Shelby's funeral, but her son, Don Hawkins, did. She died in Wichita Falls on January 25, 2011, at the age of seventy-seven.
- Ron and Jeane live in Jersey Village in a cottage behind Ron Alan's home. During the Covid-19 period of closed churches, Ron is leading a study of Navigator's 2:7 series of books on discipleship and evangelism each week. Attendees are Jeane, Ron Alan, Gail (Ron Alan's wife), grandson Brandon, Kelly (Brandon's wife), granddaughter Brittany, Kamren (Brittany's male friend), and great-grandchildren Charley and Hunter. Ron and Jeane spend prime time with eight-year-old Charley and three-year-old Hunter most weekdays.
- On November 24, 2015, M&M Manufacturing was acquired by Mitek Industries, a subsidiary of Berkshire Hathaway. At the time of the sale, M&M had two plants in Fort Worth, one each in Dallas and Houston with combined square footage of 555,300 and 750 employees compared to the one plant in Fort Worth with 4,320 square feet and 6 employees at the time Rod went to work at M&M in 1963. Rod soon joined his son Randall at Stepp Investments in Fort Worth. Mike Stepp also joined Stepp Investments a while later.
- Brandon Stepp, grandson of Ron, worked at M&M from 2012 to 2018 and was placed in inside sales during his first year. He later was transferred to outside sales and gained valuable experience and a good reputation in the air-conditioning field in southeast Texas, which prepared him for a significant sales position with Camfil who was rated the top manufacturer in the world of air filtration for the years of 2017 to 2021. Brandon was hired by Camfil in November 2018 and in 2019 doubled his 2018 M&M compensation and in 2020 tripled the same.

AN INCREDIBLE BOY AND A REMARKABLE MAN

- Jim Stepp has been retired since 1993 and lives near his daughter Meredith McClay, her husband, Mike, and their two daughters, Lily and Savannah.
- David is retired with his wife, Virginia, in Wichita Falls, Texas.
- Steve installs flooring, plays golf, and enjoys his two daughters, Sarah and Amanda, and their families. They each have three children.

APPENDIX D

Tributes to Family and Friends of Shelby

Tributes to Mother
by Ronald Lee Stepp

Ninety percent of my memories of Mother are about her working. The first is of her feeding Poofus. The second is of her washing clothes in a number 2 metal tub. The third is of her hanging out her washing. The fourth is of her sprinkling some of the clean, dry clothes with water, and then ironing them. As a two-year-old boy, I never wondered why she did not iron those washed clothes while they were wet instead of drying them first. Her regular day for washing and drying was Tuesday. She seemed to do some housecleaning every day. I do not remember Poofus and I being that messy. Poofus required three times the hours of care for a normal baby, toddler, adolescent, teenager, and adult. He was the number one priority of her life from the beginning of his birth until 1994.

She helped Daddy out at the grocery store several times a week. It seems that often she was making a dress for herself or making a pair of pants for Poofus or making a shirt for me or quilting or other. Of course, she prepared three meals each day except when we occasionally ate dinner[7] or supper at the Stepp's (our grandparents) or Ewing's (our grandparents) or Aunt Nila's or Aunt Ruth's or Bob Miller's or other. She bathed Poofus and me once or twice each week in the same tub she used for washing clothes, linens, etc., whether we needed it or not.

She took us to HHBC most Sunday mornings until we were age three and two. After that, we went to Sunday school and church most every Sunday morning, to Sunday night worship service, and to Wednesday night prayer meeting. She taught a Sunday school class. One week each summer, she taught Vacation Bible School.

Each week she took a meal to some family or took somebody to the doctor or visited a sick family member or friend or did some housework for the same.

Mother's schedule was like that for my first eighteen years. When I went off to college, she began taking in ironing to help pay for my college expenses. For five decades, Mother continued earning money by taking in ironing.

Her care for all four of her boys was unselfish, unequaled, out of a loving heart, and began each day around 6:00 a.m. and ended around 9:30 p.m. She saw that each son went off to school in clean clothes, had done their homework, and had the money for their lunch (except Shelby, she made his lunch to take to school). Shelby learned more from Mother about the meaning of life, the importance of working hard at what you are told to do, the need to respect adults who were in charge, the rewards of always doing the right thing and doing it well than he did from anyone else.

Over the many years of her life with Shelby, some found fault with her care for him. Some said she was too possessive, too restrictive, did not get more professional help in raising him and preparing him for the "real world." I never tried to determine who were making those negative statements because I did not want to know who they were. But I know one thing about them, they never walked in Mother's shoes.

---

[7] Early in the lives of Shelby and Ron, they referred to the noon meal as dinner and the evening meal as supper. Ron still does so among family and friends.

In 1994, Mother began having physical ailments that progressively reduced her ability to physically care for Shelby. After fifty-eight years of loving care unequaled by any I have seen or heard of, she was worn out. She soon began to suffer emotionally because of not being able to care for Shelby and Daddy who turned ninety in December of that year and was suffering from senile dementia, which later progressed to Alzheimer's disease. Mother always did the best she could with what she had, but she now had little left.

To me in 2021, she is the *all-time mother in the world*.

By Rod Stepp

Aunt Stella was the fourth of eleven children born to Ed and Essie Almeda Ewing. She had five brothers, Johna, Tommy, Isaac, Willie (Bud), and Harry (Boydie), and five sisters, LaVerne, Ruby, Ruth, Almeda (Sis), and Kathrine (Sonia). She and Aunt LaVerne helped their mother with cooking, cleaning, and raising their younger siblings, more than any of their siblings.

When Shelby was born, he was as crippled as anyone could be. When the doctors recommended that he be euthanized for his benefit and for Stella's benefit, she said, "God gave him to me, and I will take care of him," and she did for fifty-eight years. Never did she complain. Never did she say, "Why me?" She just took care of him the best way she could—it was as if Shelby was her major mission, her main goal.

She and Lee Roy had three more boys, and Stella was able to provide genuine care for them as well as tending to Shelby. She was a miracle worker. Of course, Shelby required more than normal attention, but somehow Stella still provided special attention to Ronnie, David, and Steve.

Stella was my aunt, but since my mother and Stella were sisters and since Lee Roy and my father were brothers, their children were more than just first cousins—they were double cousins. So, Stella was more than just my aunt, she was almost like my mother, and my mother, Ruby, was more than just Shelby's aunt, she was almost like his mother.

And since the two families shared the same house for seven years, my mother, Ruby, was able to assist Aunt Stella in the care of Shelby and his siblings.

As Shelby stated in his diary of September 12, 1995, "A part of me departed this earth at 7:30 this morning. My dearest mother left us with what appeared to be a fatal heart attack."

Saint Peter needed extra angels to assist Stella Stepp when she was ushered through the pearly gates of heaven. Her crown was so heavily ladened with sparkling jewels that she needed help to make her entrance.

Tribute to Jerry and Rita Allen
by Ronald Lee Stepp

Jerry and Rita befriended Shelby in 1965 and opened their home to him early on and left it open to him for almost forty years. Visiting family and friends in their homes was high on his list of favorite things to do. The Allen's were one of his "regulars." They were fellow active church members at HHBC for many years. Shelby enjoyed seeing them grow in Christ and take positions of service in the church. After Sunday evening church services, Shelby often enjoyed a hot dog at the Allen home. Jerry would chop Shelby's hot dog up into small pieces. He often said that his favorite meal was a hot dog.

Shelby was a batboy for the HHBC men softball team in 1965 when Jerry played third base and Ron pitched. Then he was batboy (batman) for teams that Jerry coached in kid baseball in the 1960s and 1970s. After Shelby's parents were not able to drive safely, Jerry and Rita often took Shelby shopping, to sporting events, and to other places. They gave him gifts that were needed during those later years of their long friendship.

In the mid-1970s, Jerry and Rita started focusing on volleyball, which they both played very well. A tribute to Jerry shortly after his death on December 5, 2010, is borrowed from a Wichita Falls couple:

Remembering Jerry Allen by Don and Karla Wallace

AN INCREDIBLE BOY AND A REMARKABLE MAN

We first met Jerry Allen in 1986. We first knew him as a talented and devoted vocational education teacher in WFISD. He taught auto body repair at Carrigan Center, and he directed his students as they put the last paint job on our 1968 Cougar in 1992. We learned that he grew up in Oklahoma and graduated from East Texas State University in Commerce. We knew that he was an avid volleyball player and coach who started club volleyball in Wichita Falls and coached hundreds of girls for 36 years. But we did not know him well until 2009 when he joined Wichita Christian School to coach our volleyball teams. That is when we began to really know this man of God who loved his Savior.

We fell in love with Coach Allen, and he fell in love with WCS and our students. He told his wife Rita that he would never retire from WCS because he loved it too much. None of us knew that God would call him home so soon. We are saddened at our loss, but we are so blessed that we had this short time with Coach Allen.

Tribute to Shelby's Friend
(Written by Her Grandson)

Veron Seay was not a woman people will read about in the history books. She was not famous, but she was the kind of person that the world was better for having around.

She was born Lois Veron Harris in 1927 in Ragtown, Texas, a small community of farmers just outside Paris. She had an older brother, Gaylon, who died when he was five, and a younger sister, LaFay.

The family later moved further west to Wichita Falls when she was young in hopes of better work. The Great Depression, however, hit the family hard. Her mother would have to make dresses for her and her sister out of old potato sacks. At one point, all they had to eat in the house was one can of Spanish rice. But they worked hard, endured, and gradually overcame their poverty. Family was always important.

When she was growing up, their denomination would be whatever church was within walking distance. She would go on to teach Sunday school and Vacation Bible School for nearly six decades. In 1940, she had to quit school in the eighth grade to go to work.

In 1984, she married Jeff Seay, a respected rancher and gentleman from Archer City. The two had many happy times together. Well into retirement, she continued to work. She volunteered for many years with several organizations, always helping others and always treating each volunteer job as she would any other job.

Her faith was always there, and she read the Bible and religious books regularly. Even pushing eighty, she still walked the ten blocks to and from church on Sunday mornings and Wednesday nights.

For Veron Seay, kindness, self-respect, and hard work were always a given. If someone ever took advantage of her generous nature, she would just shrug it off and move on. She would never allow someone else's lack of character to diminish her own. Being good to others was her objective in life.[8]

When her sister became ill, she cared for her day and night, refusing to leave her side. As they had been all their lives, they were inseparable. Not long after her sister passed away, her ex-husband became ill, and she took care of him too, staying at his side the whole time with all forgiven. Losing so much in the span of just a few months took its toll on Veron, and her health declined.

She was tired, but she still wanted to take care of everybody. In March, she suffered a serious stroke that briefly paralyzed her. With modern medicine and a strong spirit, she was up walking the next day. Her luck ran out, and she suffered a second stroke a month later, much more serious and one she would not be able to recover from. She died on April 16, 2016, at the age of eighty-eight.

One life touches another life. Perhaps the ultimate legacy anyone can leave is the example they lead, how they touch the lives of others, and how they made them feel. And sometimes we find a special person in our lives who makes us want to be better people. That was the special legacy of Veron Seay, my grandmother.

---

[8] Veron attended Shelby's funeral. As was stated in Shelby's diary of 1996, she had helped him complete his hoeing weeds on July 1, 1996, and she had earlier loaned her TV to him while his TV was being repaired. They were active members at HHBC at the same time for many years. They had much in common in their daily walk in Christ.

APPENDIX E

Comments by Readers of Shelby's Story

Ron, if there is a financial shortfall in publishing this book, please let me know. The joy I feel from reading it, is that I knew Shelby so well and LOVED HIS HUMOR AND RESILIENCE. It also reminds me of how determined and courageous you have been in producing this script. It also let me recall my childhood on Ave Q. All the best.

—Mickey Aboussie

Thank you, Ron. I have enjoyed reading about Shelby. Inspirational to say the least. Your dedication to tell the story of your brother is commendable. Our Lord and Savior will surely bless you and Jeane.

—Robert L. Barker

Once I started to read it, I could not put it down for two reasons. First, the strength and love and compassion of your mom and the others in your family. The determination, endurance, patience, and unexpected circumstances facing Shelby in his formative years. And second, the life of young boys growing up in Texas during that time. You give a great insight into the times and struggles and the joy of family during war and peace and the depression era and on to prosperity. I am looking forward to the next chapters."

—Ron Thorp

I finished chapter 8 and you can tell the publisher that I will buy at least 20 books to send to family and friends.

—Ron Thorp

ABOUT THE AUTHOR

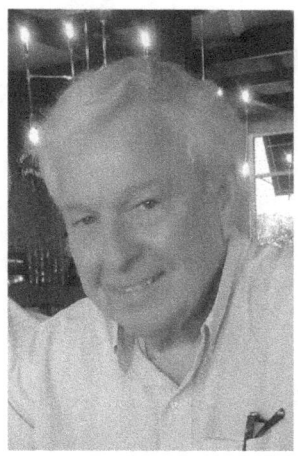

Ronald L. Stepp was born and raised in Wichita Falls, Texas. He completed seven semesters at Texas A&M University with a five-year double degree in geological and petroleum engineering. Then he enlisted in the US Army for three years and was promoted to staff sergeant two months before his honorable discharge. He was stationed in Germany during the Berlin Crisis and the Cuban Missile Crisis. He earned a bachelor of science degree in mathematics from Midwestern State University in January 1966 and began a career in the computer information systems development department of Gulf Oil and later of Chevron, providing software and databases for the geologists, geophysicists, drilling engineers, and production engineers. He visited the Abu Dhabi National Oil Company (ADNOC) to provide consultant services for their plan to develop an oil and gas well data computerized information system. After early retirement, he served as business manager at St. Christopher's Episcopal Church in Houston and then served as the minister of administration at Jersey Village Baptist Church. In the fall of 2004, he retired and with his wife, Jeane, moved to a country home they had designed and had built on Lake Livingston near Trinity, Texas. In the fall of 2017, they moved back to Jersey Village where their son, Ron Alan, lives. Their grandson, Brandon, and his wife, Kelly, and children, Charley and Hunter, also live in Jersey Village. Ronald has been an avid reader since the age of nine. He prefers biography, history, Christian, and English and American classic literature. His favorite authors are Dietrich Bonhoeffer, C. S. Lewis, William J. Bennett (also editor), Billy Graham, Sir Walter Scott, and Mark Twain. This is the first book he has written.

CPSIA information can be obtained
at www.ICGtesting.com
Printed in the USA
LVHW041023060722
722843LV00001BA/81